Best Wishes!

A Pichel

CANCER

and the

HUMAN CONDITION

Clifford S. Pukel, M.D.

Published by Cancer Vaccine Institute, LLC

Email address: cancerimmunionst@aol.com

Library of Congress Cataloging-in-Publication Date 2010
ISBN: 978-0-615-35459-0

Essays

Dedication

This book is dedicated to Lloyd J. Old, MD, a man of great vision, intellectual curiosity, and excellence of moral character.

And

To my Grandpa, Charles Buchholtz, former President of Congregation Kneses Israel, Sea Gate, Brooklyn, NY, who will always live in my heart.

All nature is but art unknown to thee;

All chance, direction, which thou canst not see...

Alexander Pope (1688-1744)
Essay on Man

Then Job answered the Lord, and said:

I know that Thou canst do every thing, and that no thought can be withholden from Thee.

Who is he that hideth counsel without knowledge?

Therefore have I uttered that I understand not;

Things too wonderful for me, which I knew not.

Hear I beseech Thee and I will speak:

I will demand of Thee and disclose Thou unto me.

I have heard of Thee by hearing of the ear:

But now mine eye seeth Thee.

Wherefore I abhor myself, and repent in dust and ashes.

Job 42:1-6

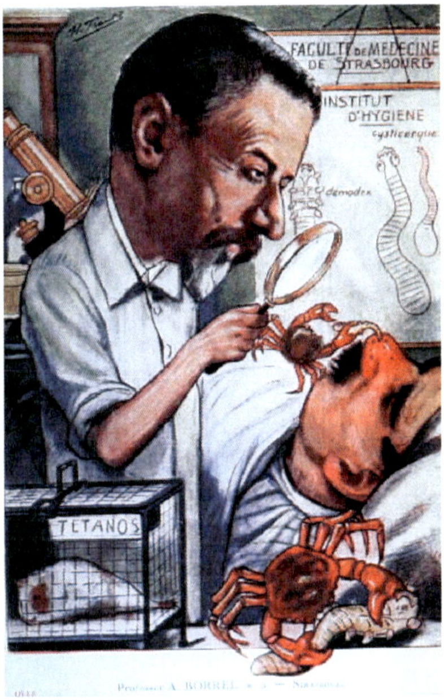

A cartoon of a 19th century cancer "expert," Dr. A. Borrel, examining a patient. More than anything else, the crab motif is a reminder of the incredible creativity of the human imagination.

Preface

If you are reading this sentence you are smart! It means the book's title and cover interested you enough to open it and I would like to think this demonstrates you have a fine mind. You may be incredibly smart (I hope so), or even a genius, but I can (within the laws of probability) guarantee you do not know more about cancer than me. Look at the odds, with 6 billion people in the world, and maybe 6 thousand cancer experts of various sorts (researchers and clinicians with many years of experience), the likelihood of one of my peers reading this is one in a million.* In fact, if the definition of an expert is: "someone who doesn't need to know anything more, otherwise they wouldn't be an expert," I doubt my colleagues will be interested in this book.

So being smart, and wanting to learn, you are already on the second paragraph. Congratulations!

As my wonderful professor of comparative anatomy, Dr. Giles McIntyre, said more than thirty years ago, "The definition of intelligence is the ability to learn, and, unlearn, if something is found to be untrue," which is precisely what this collection of essays is designed to do.

I want you to remain skeptical. I want you to be challenged, and to question the statements that are made, in a vigorous and intellectually honest way. I want you to take everything I say with a large "grain of salt." I want you to think. I want you to learn.

Much of what I say may prove to be false. It may be true today, and untrue tomorrow. That is the beauty of the scientific method.

*** I recognize that the numbers are inaccurate and the reasoning imprecise. Maybe only 1 billion people can read at all and let's not even talk about translations and accessibility to books. Odds of one in one hundred thousand may be closer to the truth.**

I am puzzled about why cancer, even the word alone, stimulates an almost visceral physical reaction in people, and their families, diagnosed with this disease. Is it the destructive changes that can occur? Is it the fear of death associated with this disease? Or is it something even more deep in the human psyche, like the notion or belief that cancer is the betrayal of self? That in other words, we have failed ourselves, in the most intimate and perhaps passionate way imaginable.

Hopefully, you will consider these thoughts as you continue your reading.

This is the first in a series of books, and I'm sure that you will have many excellent ideas about future essays.

I encourage you to share your thoughts, experiences, and reflections with us.

But for now, just open your heart and mind to ideas and images and unique connections that will inspire you, dear reader, to think about our existence in new and wonderful ways.

C. S. Pukel, MD

I. Cancer and the Human Condition*

~~ Selfishness is the greatest curse of the human race.~~
William Gladstone (1809-1898)

Cancer, like the poor will always be with us.

When I started studying cancer many years ago, I was young and idealistic, and believed that as societies evolved, with altruistic motives and with technological advancements poverty could be eliminated from this planet. In a similar fashion, and method of reasoning, I thought that cancer could also be eliminated from this planet.

I no longer believe that either of these wonderful ideas will ever be accomplished.

For there is something wrong with our species, that I think will prevent mankind from fulfilling its highest goals. The thing that is wrong with us is we are incredibly selfish. We don't like to share. We don't like others to beat us at anything; to earn more, vacation more, dress better, live in bigger or better residences, have more money, have more success, be happier, be better looking, be more popular, be smarter, be stronger.....

As we are selfish in a psychological sense, our bodies can metaphorically also be selfish. And the sine qua non of physiologic selfishness, is cancer.

Now I do not believe that selfish people by some mechanistic (or Divinely inspired) process develop selfish diseases. That is far too simplistic. But I think it is important to consider what it means when our bodies fail us in philosophically provocative ways. For, unlike other diseases, cancer, just the word alone, evokes an incredibly primitive and intense response in many people. It terrifies them. Just the word. Just the thought. Just the mental imagery. Just the idea.

* **No offense (literary or philosophical) is intended to the great social theorist and intellectual, Hannah Arendt (1906-1975), who wrote "The Human Condition", in 1958.**

This mental imagery extends to our way of responding to the diagnosis of cancer. "We are going to fight this thing." We are going to win the battle." "We are going to be cancer survivors." "We are going to defeat it.'

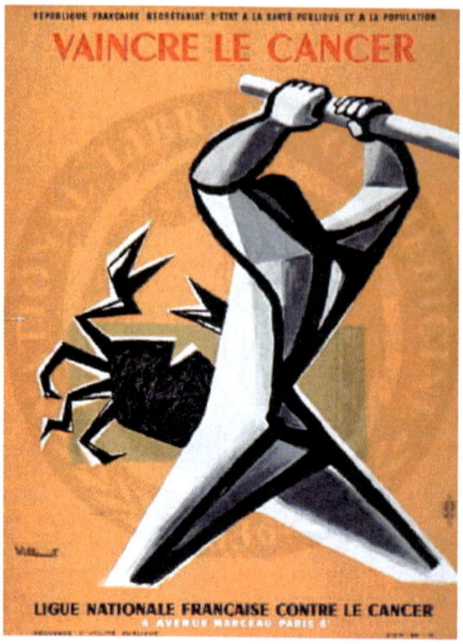
VAINCRE LE CANCER
LIGUE NATIONALE FRANCAISE CONTRE LE CANCER
"Vanquish Cancer." The eternal struggle as artistic abstraction.

So we are at war with ourselves! The battle lines are drawn. It's the good guys versus the bad guys. The bad guys, of course, are the cancer cells, that have become transformed from good guys into bad guys, so now the fight is on within ourselves.

The good guys need to be helped. So we attack the cancer with harmful drugs that will hopefully kill the bad guys without killing too many good guys, in this World War Me.

We take supplements to make our good guys work better. We meditate, pray, chant, sing, aromatize, reflexologize, all in the hope of winning. For as Vince Lombardi, the great football coach (who died of colon cancer, at age 57) said: "If winning isn't everything, why do they keep score?"

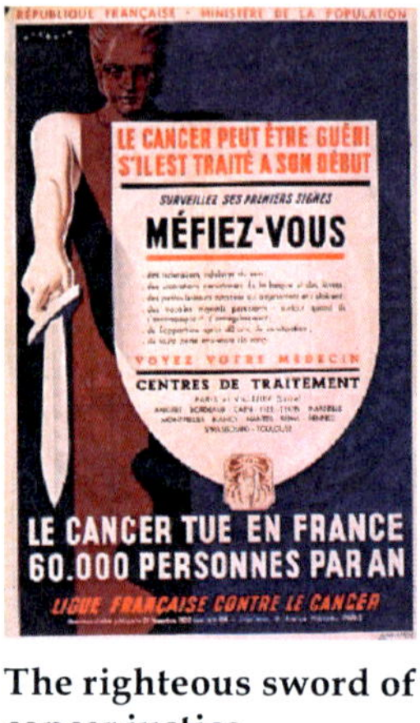
RÉPUBLIQUE FRANÇAISE - MINISTÈRE DE LA POPULATION
LE CANCER PEUT ÊTRE GUÉRI S'IL EST TRAITÉ A SON DÉBUT
SURVEILLEZ SES PREMIERS SIGNES
MÉFIEZ-VOUS
VOYEZ VOTRE MÉDECIN
CENTRES DE TRAITEMENT
LE CANCER TUE EN FRANCE 60.000 PERSONNES PAR AN
LIGUE FRANÇAISE CONTRE LE CANCER
The righteous sword of cancer justice.

I worked for several years at a Vince Lombardi Cancer Clinic, in the city where he is immortal, Green Bay, Wisconsin, and the problem is that his great success defeating football opponents did not translate into success defeating a different kind of opponent.

But consider that cancer cells, (in a special way) are as much a part of all of us as healthy cells. In other words, due to our inherent complexity as multicellular organisms, abnormal cells are created, each and every day, due to random genetic events. Since we are composed of many trillions of cells, many of which live and die as part of the normal events in cellular biology, some of these cells, just by the laws of probability, are cancer cells.

These cancer cells can do nothing or something. If they are properly recognized by the immune system, assuming it is functioning normally, they will be destroyed. Or they may, more often than not, die on their own in a process called apoptosis, which is all part of nature's design. Or they may simply remain where they are for many, many years, in a kind of suspended animation, waiting to wake up by some other stimulus, and start to cause problems. In which case they can become something. And the something they become can remain quiescent forever, very often found by accident, in an early and still nonaggressive form called in situ disease. Or the something they become can really be something, as in invasive cancer, which is typically what the layman thinks of when he or she hears the word "cancer."

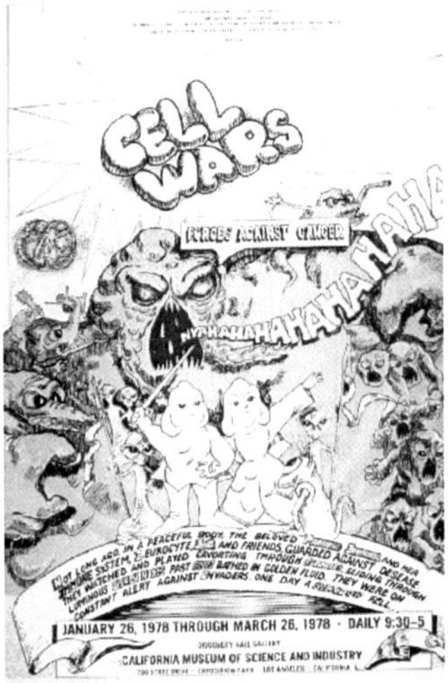

The Star Wars theme in the eternal struggle between good cells and evil cells.

Being bad, cancer cells do demonstrate a capacity to destroy us. Or kill us. Which is I suppose rarely a good thing. Although if you're 116 years old in a nursing home, bedridden, blind, deaf, sick, worn out by life, death from cancer might be considered a good thing, as long as the pain and suffering that might be part of the disease process is controlled. So the perception of cancer as always a terrible disease must be balanced by a certain realism about the human organism. Unlike taxes which may be avoided if you're incredibly rich, death (and feel free to choose the manner) is inevitable. Which reminds me of an old Yiddish saying: "If the poor could die for the rich, they would make a good living."

So when we talk about cancer, if we can avoid some of the emotional elements associated with it, perhaps more clearly. We don't talk about evil heart cells that cause heart attacks and heart failure. We don't talk about evil cells that break or clog causing strokes. We don't talk about evil pancreatic or immune cells that cause diabetes, and so on. As far as I can determine, only cancer is consistently described in such vivid and passionate ways.

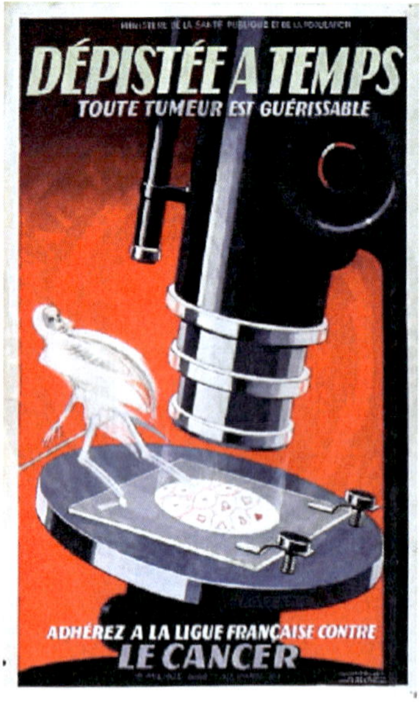
DÉPISTÉE A TEMPS
TOUTE TUMEUR EST GUÉRISSABLE
ADHÉREZ A LA LIGUE FRANÇAISE CONTRE
LE CANCER

Cancer Specter.

For cancer is evil, insidious, cruel, and destructive. Cancer is deceitful and clever as it tricks the body into thinking it is really normal. It is selfish as it grows in different places, stealing nutrients, wreaking havoc.

It betrays us, and then tries to kill us, so why shouldn't we want to attack it back, in a furious struggle of cellular good against evil.

As we continue to read these essays, perhaps it is time to reconsider the fundamental ways we speak of this disease, and treat it. I believe the relative lack of control and progress in reducing the incidence of cancer is due to an overwhelming emotion that has impaired our ability to think clearly, rationally, and scientifically about this complex disease, which is still a disease, and not a cellular football game or soap opera.

II. Forget Harvard, I Want My Kid to go to Medicare University!

~~In accordance with our principles of free enterprise and healthy competition, I'm going to ask you two to fight to the death for it.~~

Monty Python

In a free and modern society such as ours, based on democracy and capitalism, ideas which I fully endorse, there are various institutions which control the treatment of patients with cancer. The situation is complex in that typically a person cannot simply go to an oncologist and be treated with various drugs that may be helpful in controlling or curing the disease.

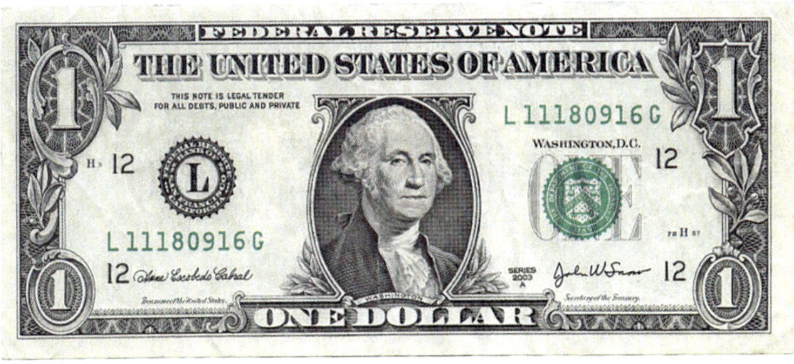

As large as this dollar bill is, as a point of emphasis, I should have probably made it even larger!

First, drugs are often extremely expensive. These drugs are created by pharmaceutical companies. These companies have employees and they want to be paid well for their labor. These companies often have shareholders who invested in stocks and want a good return on their investments. The generation of income based on so-called blockbuster drugs with sales in the billions every year, allow further drug development and so on. In our current economy it is not unusual for a drug to cost $50,000.00 a year. This cost does not include the cost of administering it, which might include hospital or clinic fees, material fees for tubing and IV fluids, pharmacy costs for drug preparation, and nursing and physician fees.

Assuming a drug has passed through the FDA (Food and Drug Administration) regulatory process, an extraordinary event in itself, somebody has got to pay for it.

If you are a billionaire, stop reading this essay. If you are of modest means and old enough or poor or sick enough to be enrolled in Medicare or Medicaid (controlled by the Centers for Medicare and Medicaid Services) (CMS), then you probably know that these government services determine to a large extent what chemotherapy or other treatments your oncologist is permitted to use, which can be translated into what treatment will be paid for. This limitation also applies to various lab tests and radiologic studies.

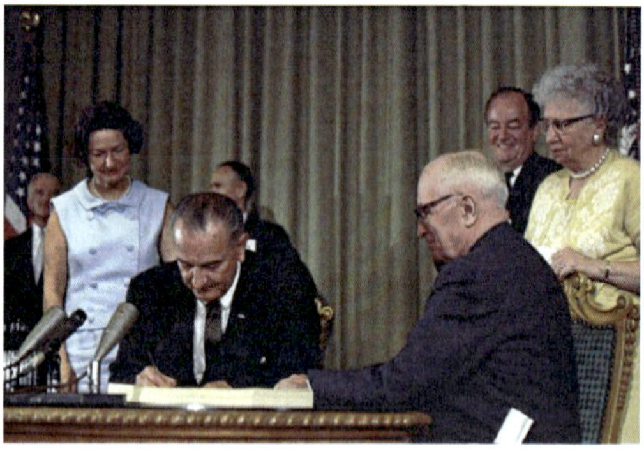

President Lyndon Johnson signing the first Medicare bill in 1965. Former President Harry Truman is sitting on the right, representing the "first" Medicare recipient. When politics dictate healthcare decisions, expect to be amazed and confused.

If a drug is not approved by CMS, it is unlikely to be approved by insurance companies. These companies also have employees and shareholders to please. For example, the recently departed CEO of United Healthcare made more than a billion dollars during his tenure.*

So outside of clinical trials that are completely paid for by the companies that are developing a new cancer treatment, which are often highly experimental and often ineffective or even dangerous, somebody has to pay.

CMS
CENTERS for MEDICARE & MEDICAID SERVICES

Confusion / Mediocrity /Silliness

* **Due to "irregularities" in the method the money was obtained, he had to give some of it back, but still made a ton of money.**

So why am I urging my kid to attend Medicare University? Because they must be the smartest people in the universe; they decide what drugs they will allow me to use in treating patients with cancer and blood diseases, for without Medicare approval with rare exception, the cost of these drugs is beyond the means of the average citizen. There is an appeals process, but despite presenting sound scientific data to support the use of non-approved drugs, including copies of papers and abstracts from distinguished academic physicians, I have had no success in reversing any decisions.

I have no idea how we can advance the treatment of cancer, while controlling costs, with the present system that exists in our country.

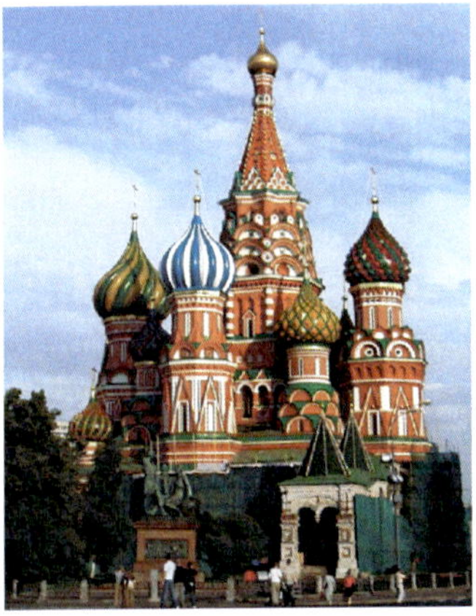

Author's conception of CMS headquarters.

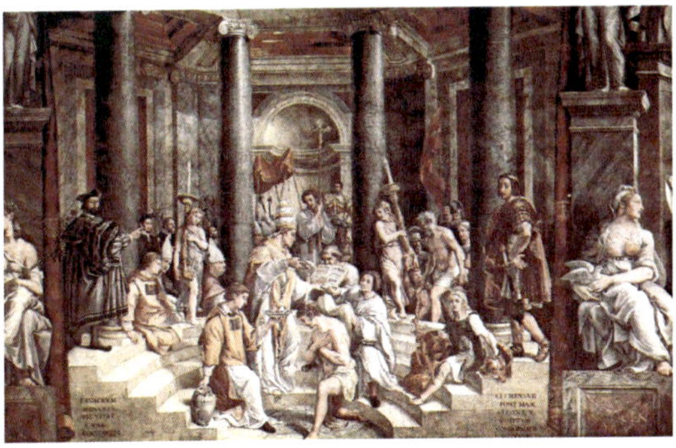

Author's conception of CMS trustee's meeting.

III. The Archer

~~Courage is being scared to death - but saddling up anyway.~~
John Wayne (1907-1979)

I think there is a way practicing physicians (and consider the word "practice" in this setting), analyze information. What I mean by this statement is that much of what we do in medicine is predicated on previous events and observations. For instance, when I see a patient with a fairly common tumor like breast cancer, I have developed a method of reasoning, after many hundreds of previous cases, which allows me to, within about a minute, figure out what to do and say. This is not to say that each case is not unique, as each patient is unique, nor that there aren't variations on a theme (which drugs to administer, participation in a clinical trial, etc.), but the basic pattern of my response is the same.

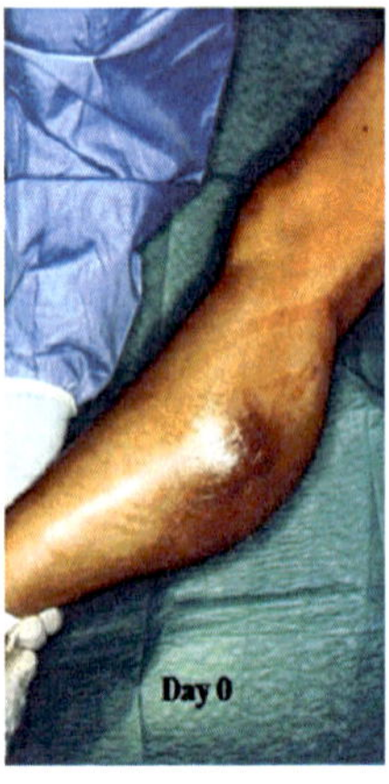

A markedly swollen red calf, representing a sarcoma similar to my patient's.

When I see an unusual or rare tumor, it's quite another thing. In fact, just the way I phrased that sentence is an indication, as I'm distancing myself from the patient, and places the emphasis on the tumor and not the person. It is interesting that when physicians speak to each other, and the way we are taught in medical school is to say something like: "This is a 25-year old man who presents with a two-year history of increasing pain and swelling in his right leg." And in the doctors' lounge: "I saw a huge chondrosarcoma today." Through a method of scientific reductionism, doctors can "simplify" a unique human being, into two sentences of information!

That's the way it is. That's the way we do things. And the rarer and more complicated the case in terms of pathology, and such, the less we care about personality or anything related to what makes us human.

Yet, when I think about this real case, seen many years ago, my mind can now reflect on different things.

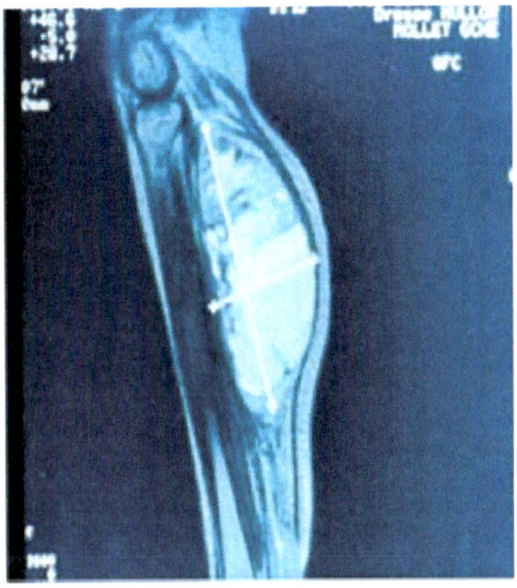

MRI scan of the leg showing a large malignant tumor similar to my patient's.

The boy came in with his mother. He was a man at 25, by only the strictest chronological criteria. At my age, a 25-year-old male is a boy. He had been in the armed forces for awhile, and the story I was told is that his right leg started to swell 2 years before, and the clinic "ran some tests and told him he didn't have a blood clot, and not to worry." So after 2 years he came to see me because his right leg, mostly around his calf muscles, was now three times the size of his left leg, and he was having trouble walking because of the pain.

There was nothing to guide me from previous experience as an oncologist, nor did we know for sure whether it was a malignant tumor as no biopsy had yet been done, so I had some time to figure things out while I sent him for an MRI scan and to an orthopedist for a consultation and tissue biopsy.

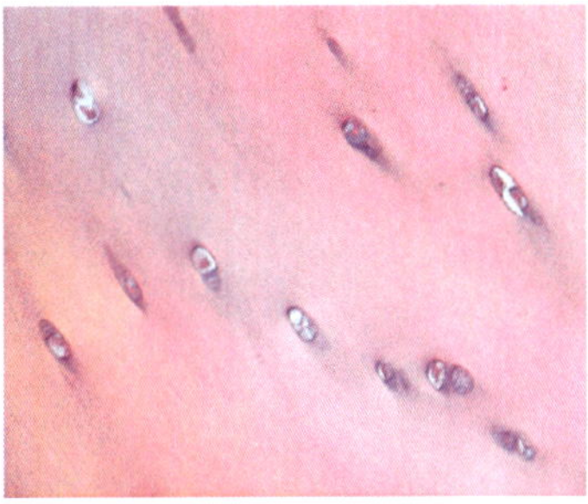

Normal cartilage cells. Notice their uniform appearance and spacing.

The following week he came back with his mother, and the pathology report was unequivocal. It was a type of cancer called a chondrosarcoma, and it was the worst kind, a so-called de-differentiated chondrosarcoma, where most of the cells in the tumor are so bizarre and abnormal, that they no longer resemble the cartilage cells from which the tumor arose. And this was a very aggressive cancer, now, as the MRI showed the tumor had replaced most of the bone and tissue of his leg, and had invaded his lymph nodes in his right groin. A CT scan also showed other sites of disease, including multiple bone and lung metastases, so this was a tough, tough situation for a young guy and his mom to deal with.

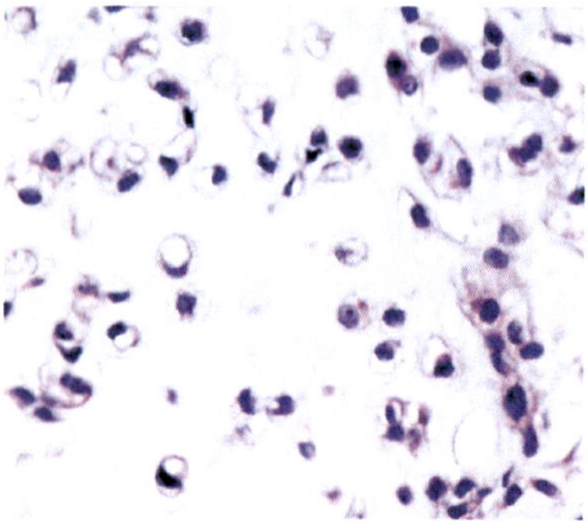

Chondrosarcoma cells. Note bizarre shapes and irregular spacing.

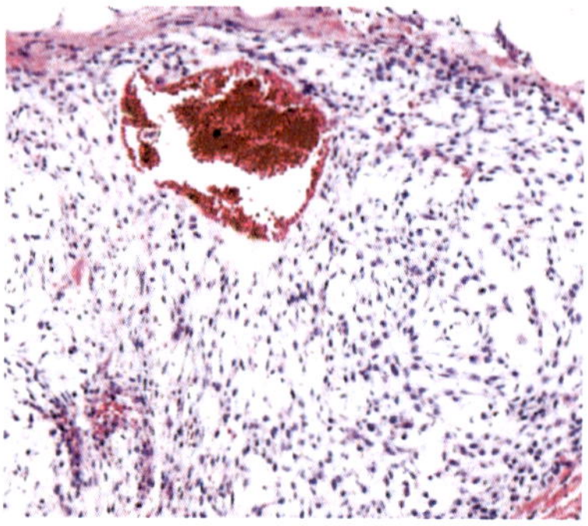

Another example of the cellular abnormalities seen in chondrosarcomas.

We talked about several options: First, whether to consider amputation of his right leg to try to decrease the tumor burden, as this was a massive tumor that might not be accessible to chemotherapy drugs or radiation, just by virtue of its incredible size and growth patterns. I was not enthusiastic about this idea, because there was still the even more ominous spread to other organs that we had to deal with and surgery first would only delay and possibly stimulate further growth of cancer at more distant sites. But, it was absolutely necessary to talk about this first, as most people reason (sometimes correctly), that surgically removing a cancer is the proper course of action, as in: "Can't you just cut it out?" Second, and perhaps more important in my way of thinking, was to consider a second opinion, and possibly treatment at a place where they see cases like this all the time. We tried to get him to the MD Anderson Cancer Center, which is a great place for this sort of case, having a large staff of oncologists who just see sarcomas. But due to financial constraints and logistics, they decided to be treated by me, and so I called one of the leaders in the treatment of these types of tumors and he recommended a chemotherapy regimen consisting of two drugs, Adriamycin and Ifosfamide (very high dose), which had been shown in clinical trials to work well about 20% of the time.

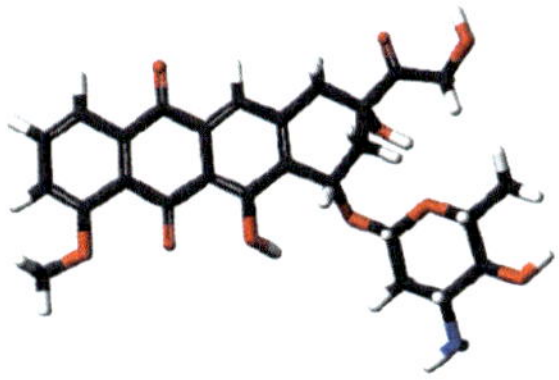

Chemical structure of Adriamycin.

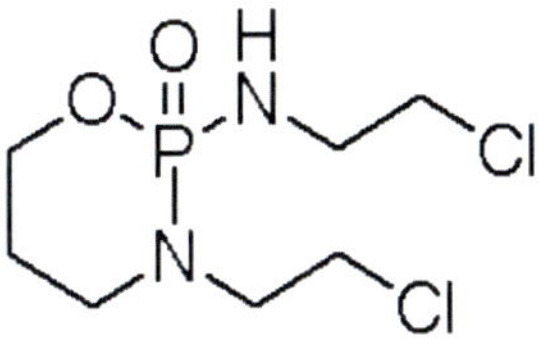

Chemical structure of Ifosfamide.

So we treated him with two cycles of chemotherapy, over about 2 months, and after the treatment, we repeated the CT and bone scans, MRI and other tests. And the cancer had now spread even further. In other words, in oncology parlance, the tumor had grown through the chemotherapy regimen, which equals disease progression, which equals an even poorer prognosis, which equals the chance that further chemotherapy would be useless. So we considered clinical trials, particularly a study at the National Cancer Institute, where if he was eligible and enrolled, all his expenses (except for transportation), would be paid for. But he was not eligible, as these studies have very specific criteria for enrollment.

Now throughout all this the boy (my initial impression) and his mom were an inspiration to me. He acted with great courage and determination, and never complained, and his mom was equally splendid in her demeanor throughout this ordeal. This was no boy; this was a man of character and excellence of spirit.

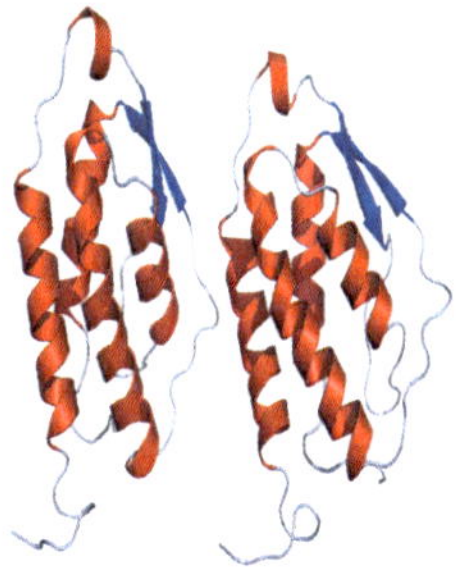

GMCSF. This complex protein can sometimes stimulate immune cells to kill cancer cells, as seen in the next image.

I told them about immunotherapy as a way of stimulating his immune system to help fight the cancer, and that with the tools available to me, the likelihood of a positive and meaningful response to treatment was very remote. But there was some suggestion that in humans the immune system could recognize sarcoma-related antigens, and maybe we could get lucky in stimulating it to do better and control his disease for awhile, and in the meantime keep exploring possible new treatments that might be available in the future. They recognized that the treatment might cause an earlier death or other bad outcomes, and we were always very honest and realistic about the disease and the limits of both conventional and experimental therapy.

I tried injecting the primary tumor in his leg and another easily accessible site of disease that had developed on his back, during chemotherapy, with three different substances that had some immunostimulatory properties, Interferon alpha-2b, interleukin-2, and GMCSF (granulocyte-macrophage colony stimulating factor), all of which were FDA approved for other uses, so this would represent what is called in medicine, "off-label use."

We repeated all the scans before starting immunotherapy and by then the cancer appeared to be growing in his lungs with multiple ball-like lesions and large collections of fluid which appeared to represent what are called bilateral malignant effusions. Nothing happened to the primary tumor or subcutaneous metastasis as I injected them about once a week, but after 6 weeks of treatment, I repeated all the scans and to my absolute shock, amazement, and general disbelief, the lung CT showed essentially no disease! Other weird things occurred like what appeared to be a sclerotic-type process in some of the bones that had disease before and areas of sclerosis in some areas of the primary leg tumor.

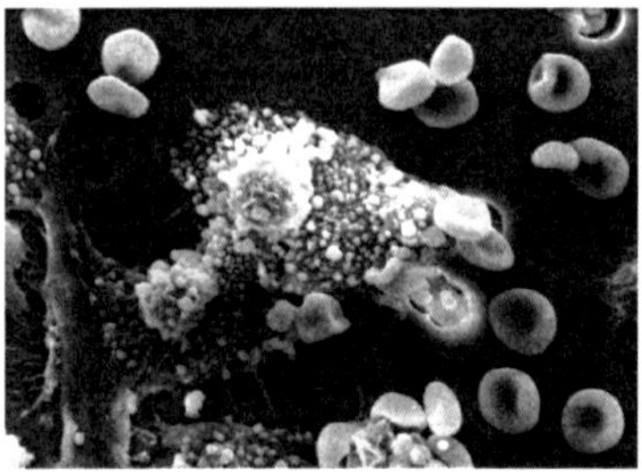

Macrophages can be activated with cytokines like GMCSF to kill cancer cells.

Despite this incredible and mysterious event (possibly the result of stimulating the immune system and other cells), the man continued to lose weight and repeat studies after four weeks showed the lung lesions still nearly all gone or "resolved," but soon after they returned and eventually the cancer won, despite our best efforts.

I sent my case report to be reviewed by people I thought would be interested in my observations. Nothing ever came of it from a scholarly perspective, nor was I encouraged to pursue things by my employers at the time. I believe something meaningful happened that may be worth investigating further in the future, with more specific adjuvants and immunotherapy drugs than I used.

I can still see this wonderful young man in my mind, and will always think of him as an extremely courageous person who dealt with a terrible disease in an almost Biblical manner. For he loved archery above all things. And I leave you with this quote from Genesis, in which Jacob (or Israel), near death blesses his sons, each in a unique and beautiful phrase. For his son Joseph, who had suffered so greatly, but never lost faith, and eventually became as great as his father.

"Joseph is a fruitful bough, even a fruitful bough by a well; whose branches run over the wall: The archers have sorely grieved him, and shot at him, and hated him: But his bow abode in strength, and the arms of his hands were made strong by the hands of the mighty God of Jacob..."(1)

A promise kept to a brave archer, Clifford Cook, whom I will always remember.

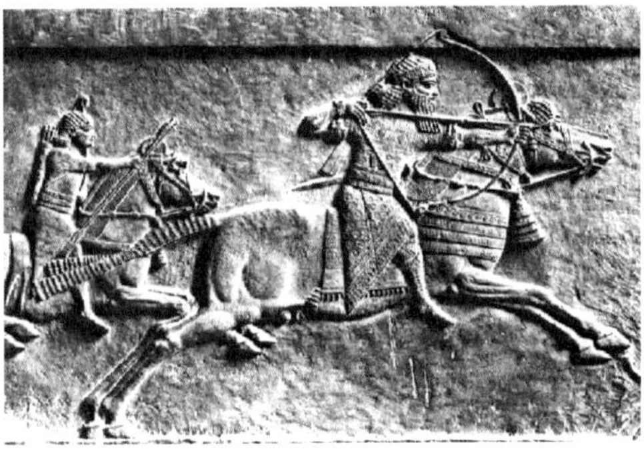

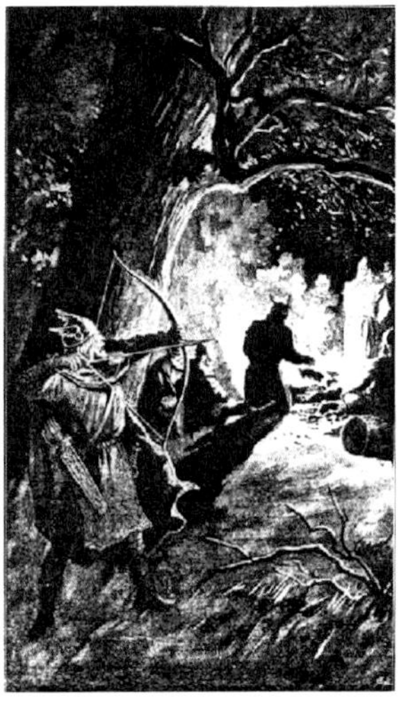

Heroic archers.

IV. The Chronicle of Death

~~There are three kinds of lies: lies, damned lies, and statistics.~~
Benjamin Disraeli (1804-1881)

The American Cancer Society has published its annual report on global cancer. This report can be accessed online for interested readers (www.cancer.org) by looking under cancer facts and figures.

The number of new cancer diagnoses worldwide is more than 12 million.* This number excludes common skin cancers (squamous cell or basal cell) which number in the millions by themselves!

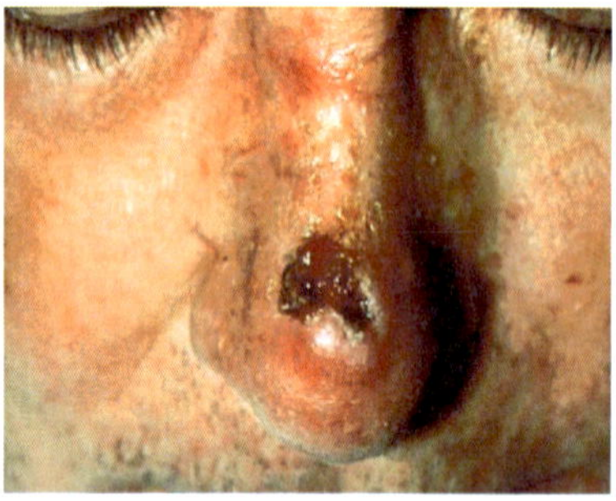

Squamous cell carcinoma.

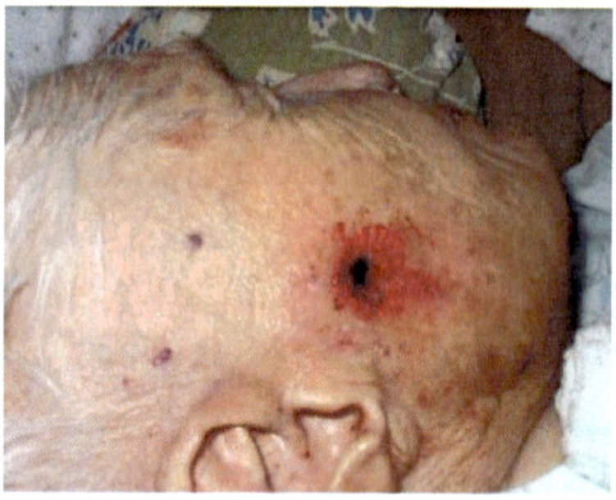

Basal cell carcinoma.

It seems incredible that cancer registries do not even include these types of cancers, which number in the millions, in their data collection.

What these staggering numbers truly represent is the topic of this essay, and the perfect opportunity to talk briefly about cancer statistics. When scientists talk about the incidence of cancer they are generally referring to the number of new cases discovered over a period of time (i.e. per year). The prevalence of cancer refers to cases that have already been identified and are still alive. Therefore the prevalence of cancer is a much higher number than the incidence as people can live with cancer for many years.

When physicians talk to patients with cancer, they often discuss their prognosis. This is typically translated in layman's terms into how long they are expected to live. Different quotes

* **Figures from 2007 with similar numbers in 2008 and 2009.**

may be heard and, beyond being scientifically invalid, are sometimes incredibly mean-spirited and idiotic, such as, "My doctor told me I had 3 months to live with no treatment and 6 months with treatment." These statements strike terror and fear into the hearts of patients and their families. And they are false. The prognosis for any particular person with cancer is entirely unknown except to God Almighty. If He speaks to someone with cancer, that's a different story. If your doctor tells you have X number of months to live, take what is said with considerable skepticism.

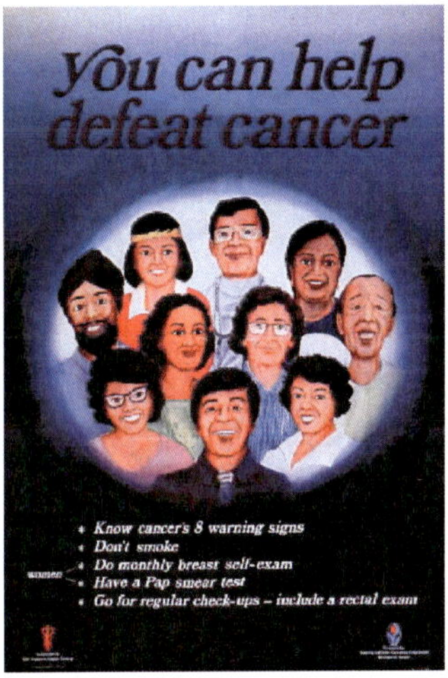
You can help
defeat cancer
Know cancer's 8 warning signs
Don't smoke
Do monthly breast self-exam
Have a Pap smear test
Go for regular check-ups – include a rectal exam

An imposible expectation fueled by irrational reasoning.

What we can talk about in scientific terms is how long a population can be expected to live or not. In other words individual survival can never be accurately predicted, but if you took a 1,000 people with a similar tumor, stage, age and other health problems, their survival could be predicted. I assure you, within that population some individuals will live way beyond our expectations (statistically) and other people will unfortunately die much sooner than expected.

Despite spending trillions of dollars over many decades, the world can expect cancer statistics to remain fairly constant over time.

Political and social institutions will continue to encourage us to decrease our risk of cancer by not smoking, eating better, seeing your doctor, exercising, and such, but I predict the numbers will not change dramatically. In fact, we should expect the cancer prevalence rate to increase over time, with better treatments.

As you continue reading this book, the reasons for all of this will become clearer, just be patient.

V. Your Grandmother was Right!

~~Give a man a fish, and you'll feed him for a day. Teach a man to fish, and he'll buy a funny hat. Talk to a hungry man about a fish, and you're a consultant.~~ Scott Adams (1957-)

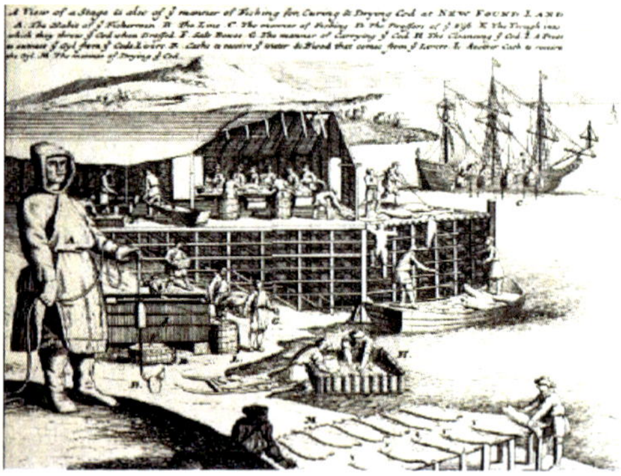

Codfish industrialists in the 18th century.

If you wait long enough the scientific pendulum swings back. This may be particularly true in what some might consider to be "old wives tales." The story begins a few hundred years ago when Norwegian fishermen started to ingest Cod liver oil to protect against the cold and illness. It tasted terrible so it must be good for you, and children were given it despite their protests.

Well guess what? Cod liver oil is a great source of Vitamin D and Vitamin A. Vitamins as a class of chemicals act typically as coenzymes in biochemical reactions critical for life. With specific attention to Vitamin D, its deficiency in childhood causes rickets, and in adults, osteoporosis.

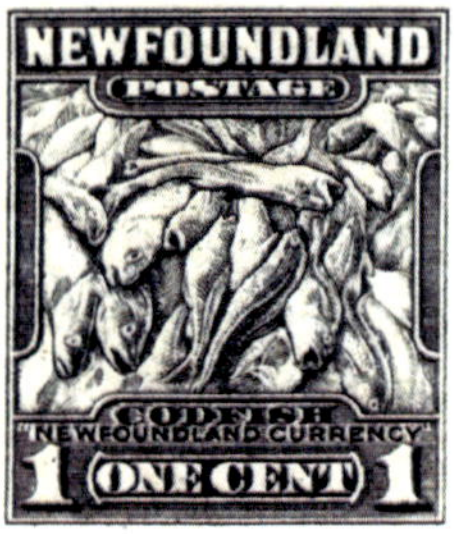

How many fish have a stamp created for them?

But these are things we all know.

But how about Vitamin D (and its analogs) as a treatment for cancer? I just treated a man with metastatic protate cancer today with calcitriol which is a Vitamin D derivative. Together with Taxotere, calcitriol seems to improve response rates and survival compared with Taxotere alone. (2)

And how about Vitamin D as a cancer prevention drug? There is good evidence that the risk of colon, breast, prostate, and ovarian cancer can be lowered by adequate Vitamin D intake (probably around 1000 IU/day). (3, 4)

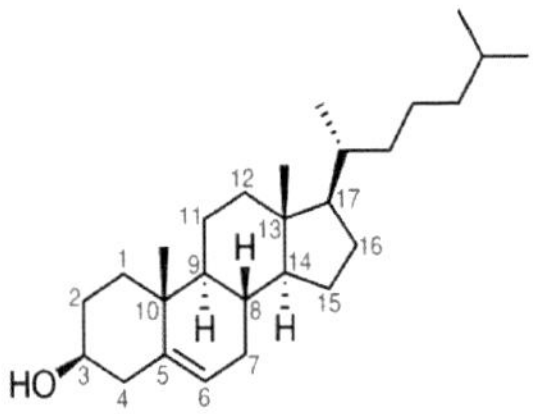

Cholesterol

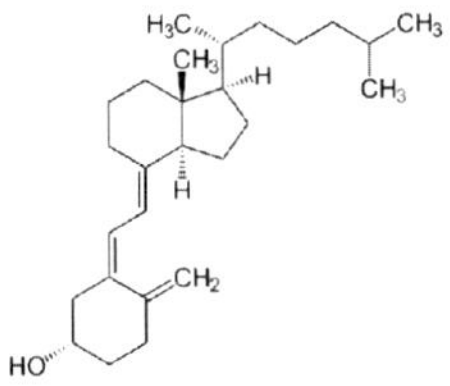

Cholecalciferol

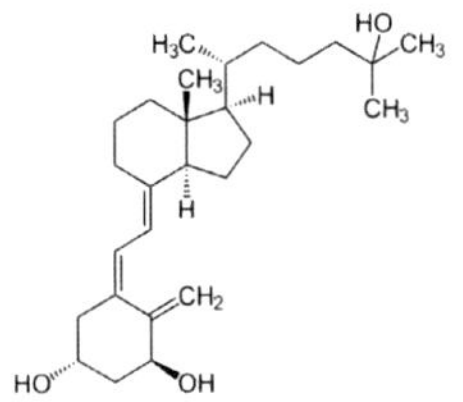

Calcitriol

Note the similarity in structure between cholesterol (which is synthesized into vitamin D) and the vitamin D analog calcitriol used in treating prostate cancer.

The mechanism of action may be related to Vitamin D (which is synthesized in the skin from a cholesterol derivative) acting as a hormone and binding to a Vitamin D receptor, which then becomes activated and influences other biochemical pathways in cells. (5)

So a tablespoon of Cod liver oil has about 1,300 IU of Vitamin D, which may be the highest naturally occurring source of this vitamin on earth! But don't just rush out to buy some or to go fishing in the North Atlantic.

Be careful to check to see that the Vitamin A content is not too excessive, as too much Vitamin A can be very toxic. In fact, people have died from Vitamin A poisoning when they ate polar bear livers (don't ask me why they were eating polar bear). So before taking: read the label of Cod liver oil preparations carefully (which come in capsule form also) and ask your doctor or pharmacist about drug interactions that might occur.

Now consider this journal article title: "Could ultraviolet B irradiance and Vitamin D be associated with lower incidence rates of lung cancer?" (6) As you already know, Vitamin D is made in the skin from a cholesterol precursor. But to make this happen the body needs a certain amount of sunlight exposure and without it Vitamin D levels are too low, which may increase the risk of lung cancer along with the other cancers mentioned. Vitamin D levels (in the form of 25 hydroxyvitamin D) can be measured in the laboratory if you are concerned about your level being too low.

So a teaspoon or so of Cod liver oil a day may keep cancer away! And to speculate a bit, I wonder whether the rate of cancer being much lower 100 years ago, might be due in part to the liver of the lowly Cod!

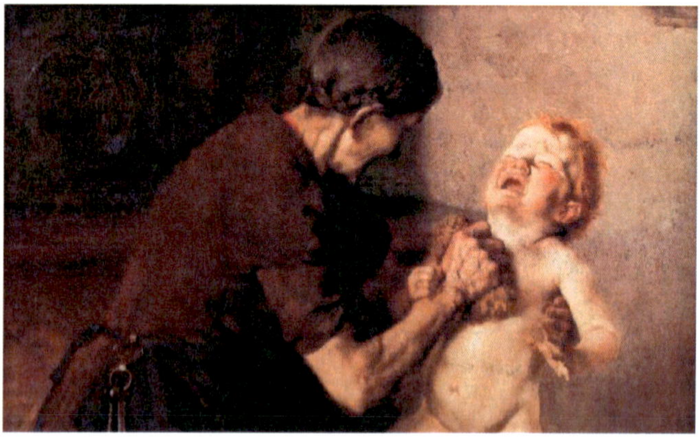

Precious moments with Grandma.

VI. Let Us Now Praise Famous Dogs

~~ If I have any beliefs about immortality, it is that certain dogs I have known will go to heaven, and very, very few persons.~~

James Thurber (1894-1961)

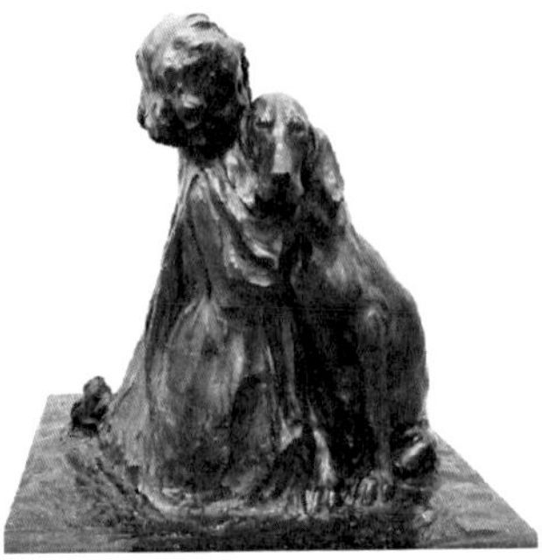

No greater love.

The dog has been domesticated for thousands of years and has shared much of recorded history with their human masters. This incredible social intimacy continues unabated to this day. In fact beyond the love and affection that they provide, they have served us in other less apparent ways that deserve our deepest respect.

I remember 35 years ago when I was a student at Memorial Hospital/Sloan Kettering Institute, an image that was truly profound. It was a scene that I cannot forget, of a hospital gurney with white sheets and attendants that one sees in hospitals all the time, but on it was a dog that had been intubated and was being wheeled away from and operating room.

I have no idea what the dog was doing there and whether it was simply an experimental animal (which I suspect but cannot confirm) used for whatever purposes that animals are used in research.

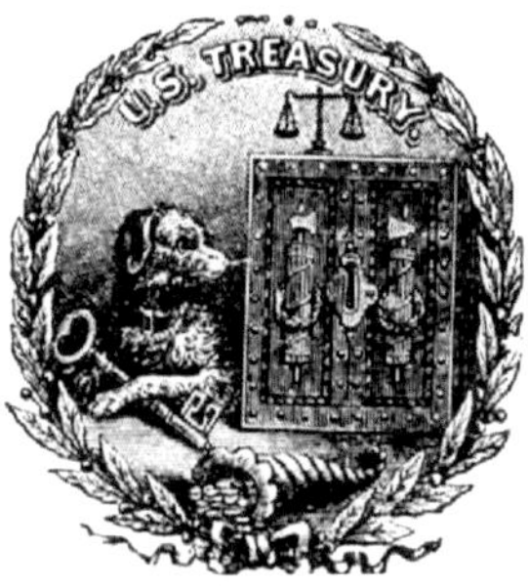

Seal of the United States Treasury Department, circa 1800.

But the dog has always been willing to risk its life for mankind, and it is a great truth that these domesticated wolves, with all their wonderful variation in form, temperament and function, are "man's best friend."

My wife and kids have 5 dogs, Lima, Oprah, Annie, Honey, and Bianca.* We also have cats and other critters (we'll talk about cats another time.)

* **Poor little Bianca, a Shitzu-Australian Shepherd mix died unexpectedly before this book was published. We all miss her terribly.**

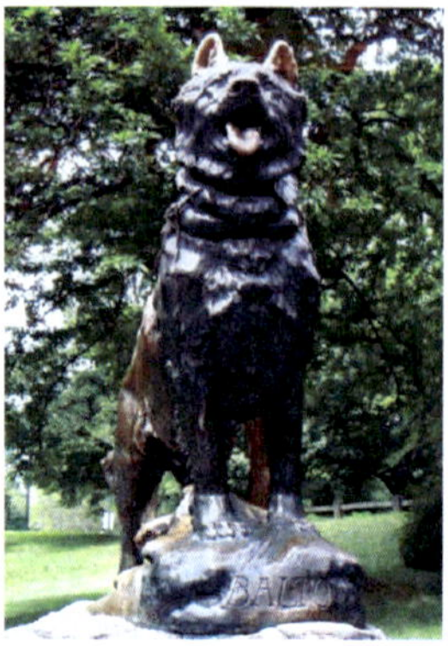

Balto: Greatness of spirit.

We love our dogs. Each unique in personality and capacity and above all their love. Each capable of expressing their love and devotion in ways that touch our hearts and souls.

In Central Park in New York City there is a statue of Balto, a sled dog that helped save hundreds of children from possible death during a Diphtheria epidemic in Nome, Alaska in 1925.

There was Marjorie, a dog that sacrificed itself to help Dr. Frederick Banting, and his medical student Charles Best, isolate insulin, which is necessary for many diabetics to live, and in so doing, in the 1920's, saved countless thousands of lives of patients with Type 1 diabetes; for before then, that diagnosis meant certain death.

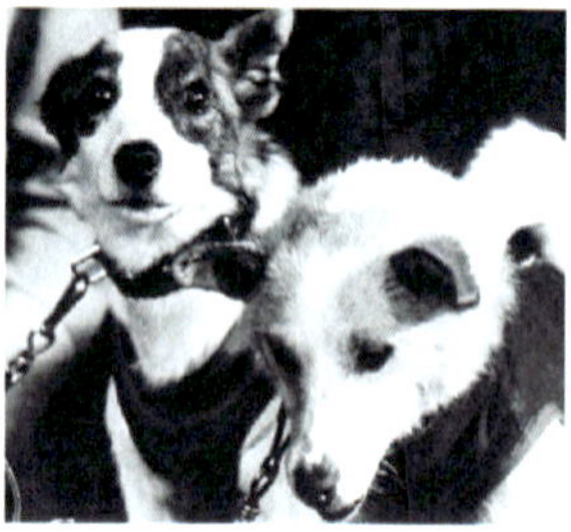

Belka & Strelka: Brave Soviet comrades.

There were Belka and Strelka, Russian cosmonaut dogs, who explored outer space in Sputnik 5 before any man.

In 2005 another hero, Tasha, who with only blood samples, allowed scientists to complete the genetic sequence of the dog genome (www.genome.gov/17515860) (7). As a result, we will be better able to understand the genetics of cancer.

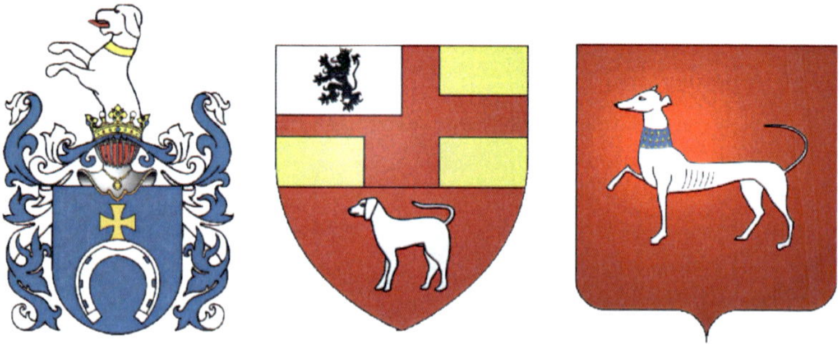

Coat of arms as a sign of nobility.

There was Hildegarde, our German Shepherd, who died 3 years ago at the age of 10, after battling inflammatory breast cancer for 2 years. My heart is still broken, for I could not save her despite two surgeries and a trial with tamoxifen. Despite her suffering, she was always a great friend.

What I learned was yet another lesson in sadness and humility. But think of the magnificent dignity of these wonderful creatures; of such goodly souls! So we endure, and suffer, and keep trying to penetrate the mysteries of life and death.

So when I heard about a cancer vaccine recently approved for dogs with malignant melanoma, a disease I studied for many years at Sloan Kettering Institute in the laboratory of Dr. Lloyd Old, one of the world's greatest cancer immunologists, I was particularly intrigued.

This vaccine is a most improbable success. Created by Dr. Jedd Wolchok and his colleagues at Memorial Hospital and the Animal Medical Center, it is derived from the DNA of melanoma cells that produce an enzyme that is often overproduced and abnormal in these tumors called tyrosinase. (8)

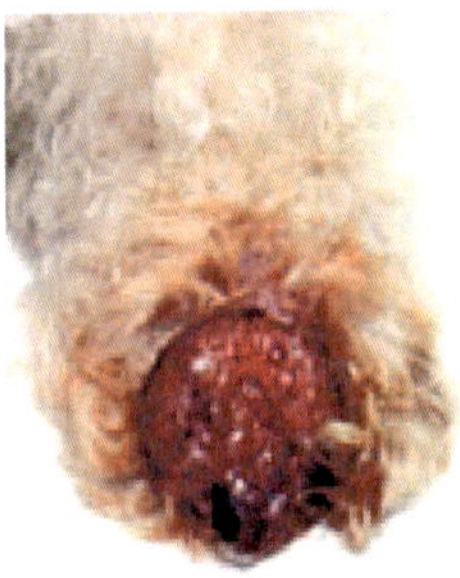

Dogs and humans share many cancers, including malignant melanoma. This is a nonpigmented (amelanotic) type in a poor little dog's paw.

By injecting this DNA into dogs with malignant melanoma that would often kill them within weeks, many dogs had their tumors, which had been widespread, disappear completely for months or even years. Some were even cured.

This vaccine has been approved by the US government for use, and could save or at least prolong the lives of many thousands of our best friends. Other canine cancer vaccines are being developed (one estimate is that 4 million dogs get cancer every year), and we will learn much about treating human cancer in this way.

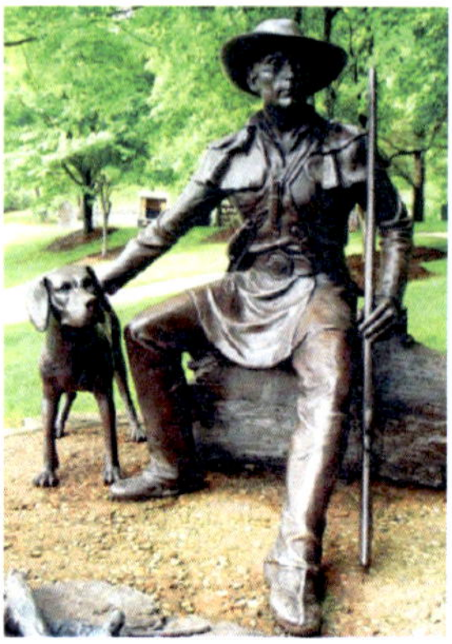

Daniel Boone & his dog.

But the ironic twist to all this is that the DNA injected into these poor animals, that helps them fight cancer and live longer, happier lives, is derived from his grateful master, man!

So to celebrate our German Shepherd Honey's second birthday today, I leave with a poem, nearly forgotten, written more than 400 years ago, by Sir John Davies:

Thou sayest thou art as weary as a dog.
As angry, sick, and hungry as a dog.
As dull and melancholy as a dog.
As lazy, sleepy, idle as a dog.

But why dost thou compare thee to a dog?
In that for which all men despise a dog.
I will compare thee better to a dog.

Thou art as fair and comely as a dog.
Thou art as true and honest as a dog.
Thou art as kind and liberal as a dog.
Thou art as wise and valiant as a dog.

VII. The Broken Clock

~~The trouble with our times is that the future is not what it used to be.~~
Paul Valery (1871-1945)

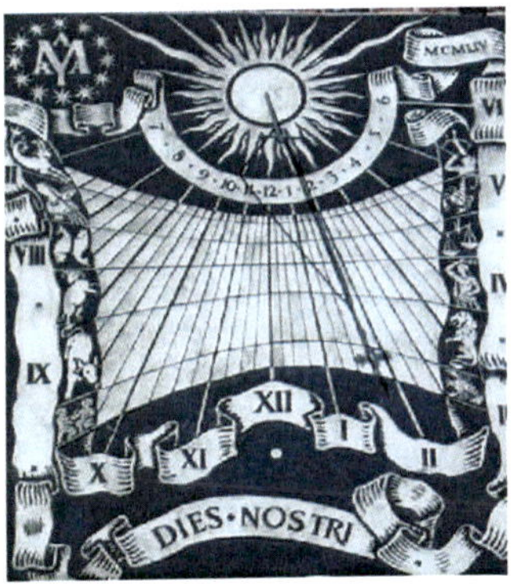

A sundial may not be accurate on a cloudy day.

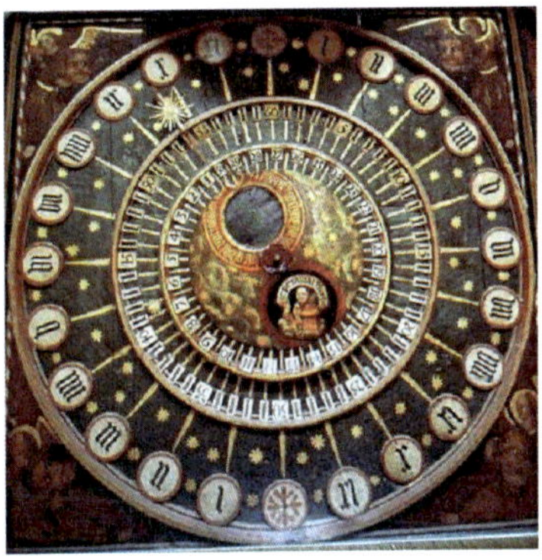

Difficult to rewind.

With the discoveries made by Albert Einstein, we know that time is relative. The way we experience time is to some extent subjective (assuming we are not traveling near the speed of light), so for instance, when you are being nagged by your spouse, or at a boring lecture, or reading something that seems like it's endless and going nowhere, or waiting in traffic, or waiting in line, or...

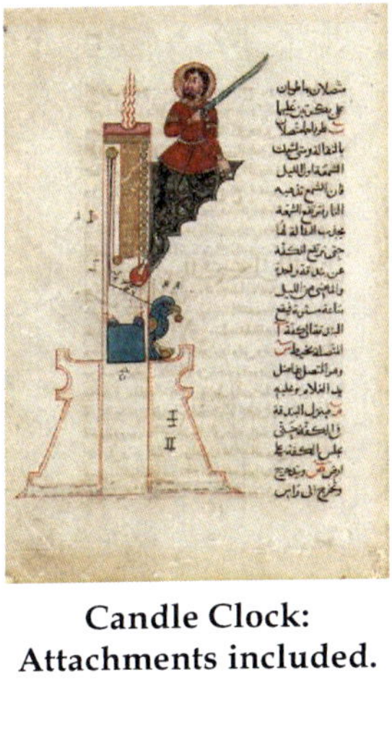

**Candle Clock:
Attachments included.**

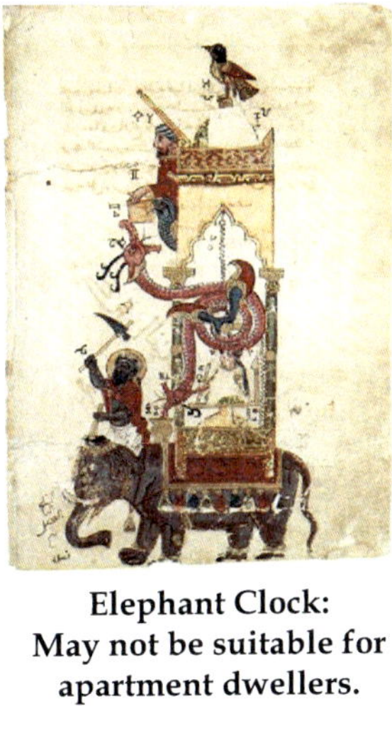

**Elephant Clock:
May not be suitable for apartment dwellers.**

Or watching a beautiful sunset, or dreaming of the most beautiful girl in the world (or boy)... Or reading this essay!

So sometimes a minute seems like an hour and sometimes an hour seems like a minute.

And sometimes something or someone belongs to an earlier time, and so we call this an anachronism. There is even a Society for Creative Anachronism, with 30,000 members throughout the world who pretend to be personalities in the Middle Ages and Renaissance, and they (as I discovered) will wrap your holiday book purchases at Barnes & Noble bookstore, in Madison, Wisconsin!*

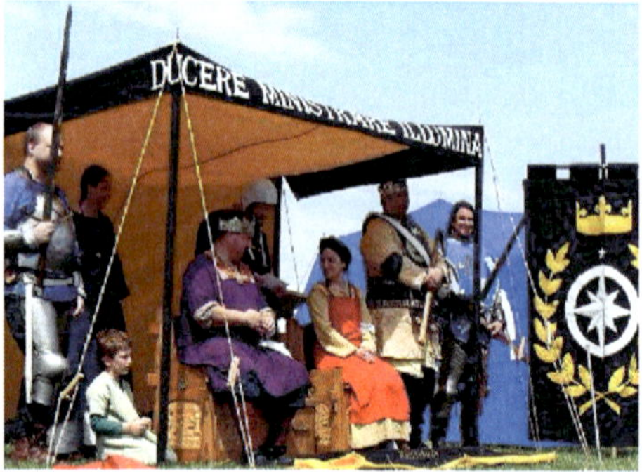

When not at court or in combat, Nobles may be found wrapping holiday books for the commoner.

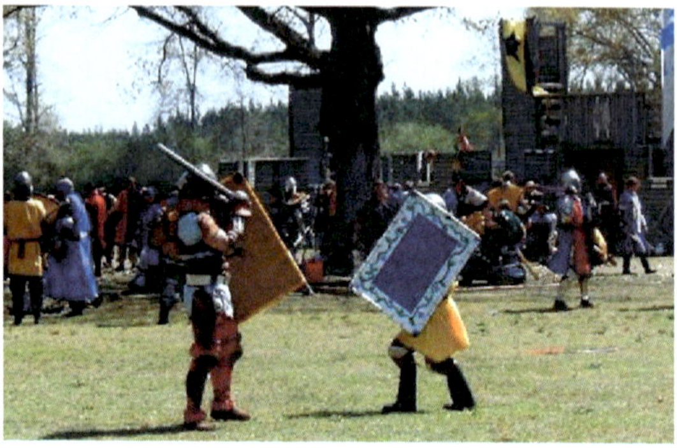

Before you give up on the relevance of this discussion (for after all shouldn't we be talking about cancer and blood diseases, or at least medical research?), consider the Sweet Clover plant.

*** I've seen them, costumes and all, in the Gulfport, MS, Barnes & Noble, too!**

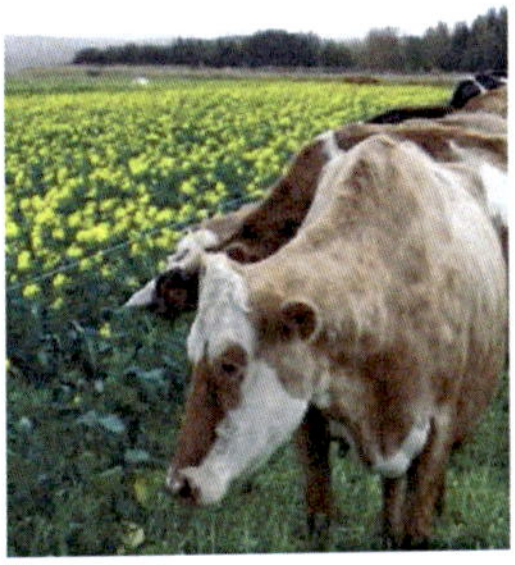

Ruminant's delight!

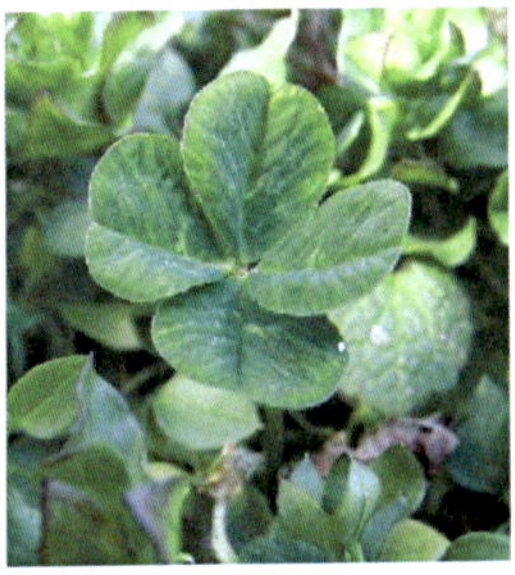

Is a moldy 4-leaf clover still lucky?

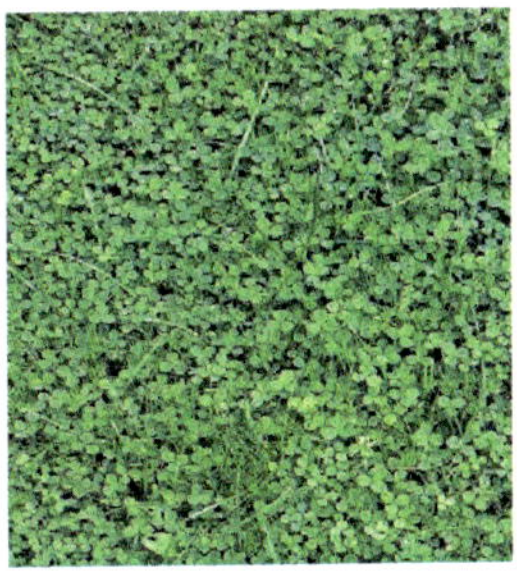

Delicious when fresh.

Cows in Wisconsin (The Dairy State) eat plants. The Sweet Clover sometimes becomes moldy. Cows in general don't care about a little mold and eat it anyway. But when they eat too much they get sick, and bleed from their nose and mouth spontaneously and sometimes even die from massive hemorrhage. This was something that, of course, upset farmers, who told veterinary doctors, who talked to chemists, who eventually isolated a compound in 1940 from this moldy plant.

The chemist, Dr. Link, and his student were on the faculty of the University of Wisconsin, in Madison. So they called this substance warfarin (Wisconsin Alumni Research Foundation... arin). Most people call it Coumadin now, but it's the same chemical. As the story goes, after a US Navy sailor in 1950 tried to overdose (by ingesting rat poison) (and lived) someone thought of the idea of using rat poison (warfarin) in treating people at risk for blood clots and heart attacks.

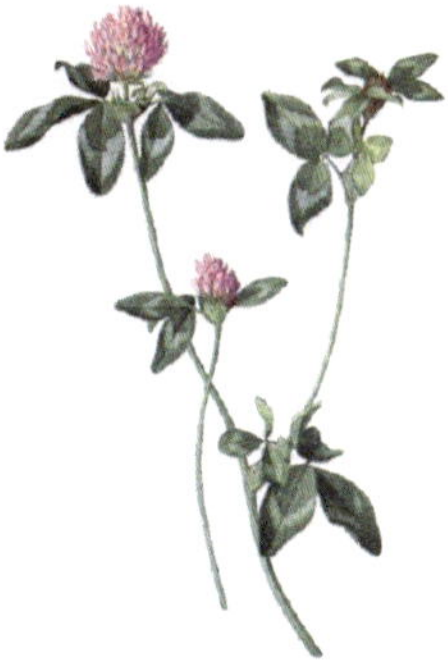

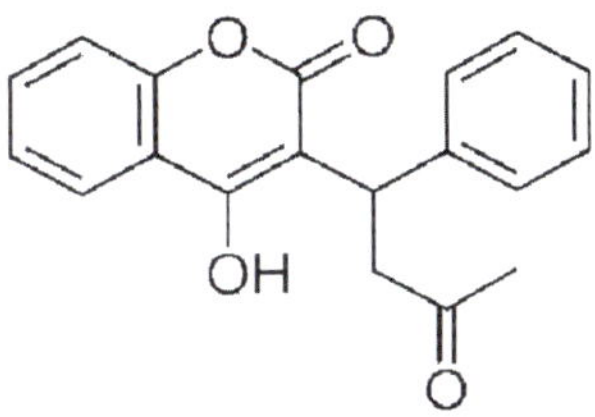

Who would imagine that Coumadin was derived from a moldy plant?

Another substance isolated from pig and cow intestines and other tissue is called heparin, and it was first discovered in 1916 by Dr. McLean and his student at Johns Hopkins University. Heparin is a complex sugar molecule called a glycosaminoglycan which also has tremendous utility in treating people with or at risk for blood clots and has also saved the lives of countless cancer patients through the years, as cancer often increases the risk of blood clots which can often migrate to the lung, an often fatal complication called a pulmonary embolus.

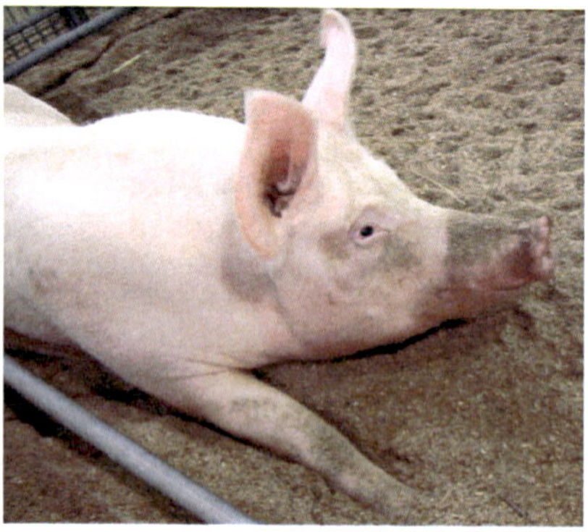

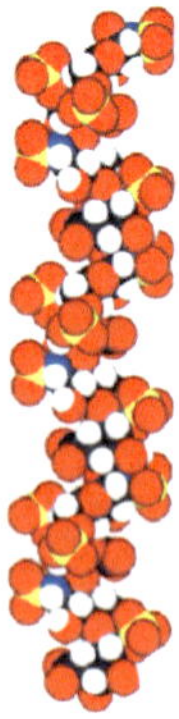

Heparin is now usually derived from pig intestines.*

But what does this have to do with anachronisms? Well, consider the leech.

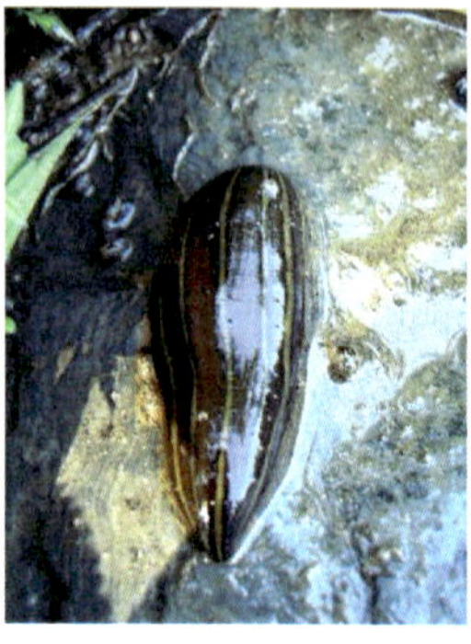

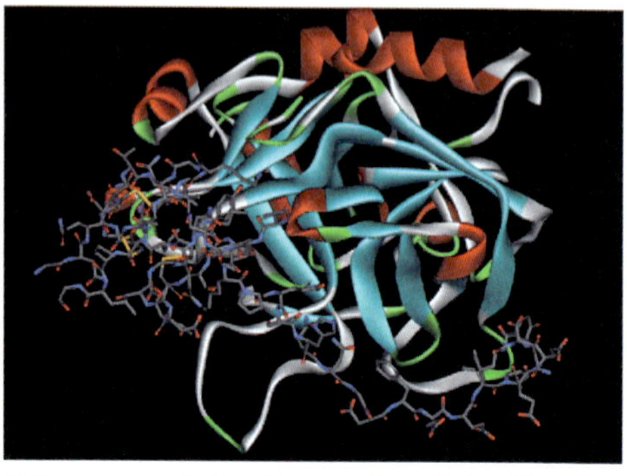

The yucky leech, source of the powerful anticoagulant hirudin, shown in combination with thrombin, a molecule that when uninhibited, promotes blood clots.

*** Most heparin worldwide is initially derived from Chinese manufacturers. Lack of FDA oversight at these foreign plants has recently led to a number of deaths from contaminated preparations. A congressional investigation is underway at the time of this writing. Ref: FDA website news update 4/21/08.**

For thousands of years doctors have used leeches to remove blood from patients. And they're still using them in plastic surgery in selected cases in 2008!

For the leech produces an anticoagulant called hirudin which is present in the critters' saliva. A few years ago it was approved for use in patients at risk for blood clots. It is a genetically produced version of leech spittle called lepirudin and it is useful in people who cannot tolerate heparin-like substances or Coumadin. And there are many other anticoagulant molecules in various stages of development soon to be available.

Our anachronistic list includes a method of treating blood diseases such as hemochromatosis and Polycythemia vera (Osler-Vaquez disease).

Now these diseases can be identified by a simple blood test that detects the gene mutation associated with each disorder. This is high-tech stuff and in fact the definitive studies on Polycythemia vera (P. vera) were not published until 2005 (9, 10).

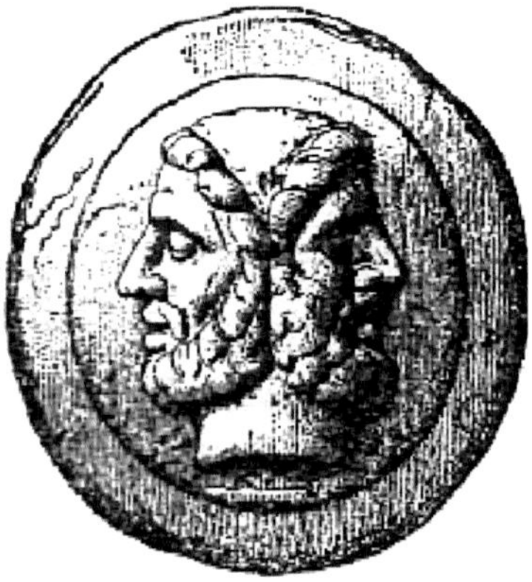

Janus – Roman god now named for a type of enzyme.

So with P. Vera we now know that in this type of myeloproliferative disorder (associated with overproduction of red blood cells in the bone marrow, which are released into the bloodstream) most cases are caused by an abnormal genetic mutation in the JAK2 (Janus kinase) gene which creates an abnormal protein.

Janus, the Roman god of doorways and gates had two faces and he is still remembered by molecular biologists. But this is not anachronistic enough for us, nor have we tied together the theme of this essay.

For since Cain and Abel, the spilling (or removal) of blood has had a profound influence on human history.

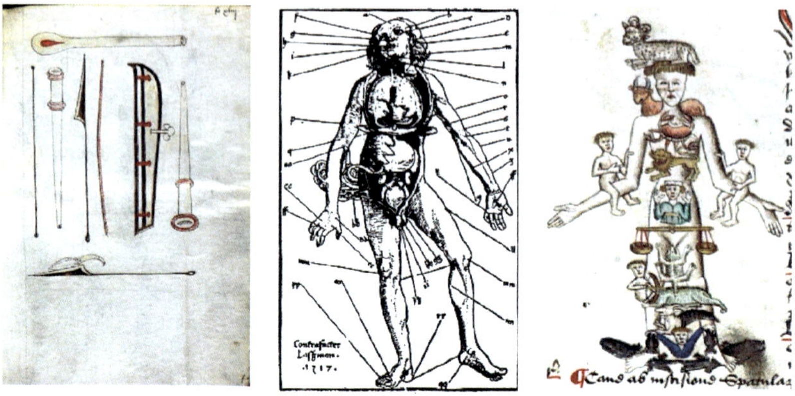

Medieval surgical and bloodletting instruments along with easy-to-follow instructions to remove blood from diferent sites, depending on the disease. Ouch!

Besides the leech and lancet, a number of instruments have been used to remove blood from people. The medical term now is therapeutic phlebotomy. But the result of this "therapy" has been almost universally disastrous, killing and injuring people by removing large amounts of blood from them for incorrect reasons. The pervasive belief until the 19th century was that by removing blood (one of four essential substances called humours, the others being black bile, yellow bile, and phlegm), doctors could alter the imbalance that caused various diseases. Even personality was directly attributed to these qualities or temperaments, hence; sanguine, melancholy, choleric, and phlegmatic.*

George Washington, our beloved President on the dollar bill, was essentially killed by his physicians when he was bled a couple of quarts of blood for a sore throat.

When is a broken clock not broken?

Even a broken clock is right twice a day. And in treating hemachromatosis and Polycythemia vera, bloodletting is the absolute correct treatment, which is as true today as it was 3,000 years ago. As for the unnecessary and deadly treatment of nearly everyone else, as we say in medicine... oops!

VIII. Bric-a-Brac

~~Be not forgetful to entertain strangers for thereby some have entertained angels unawares.~~ Hebrews 13:2

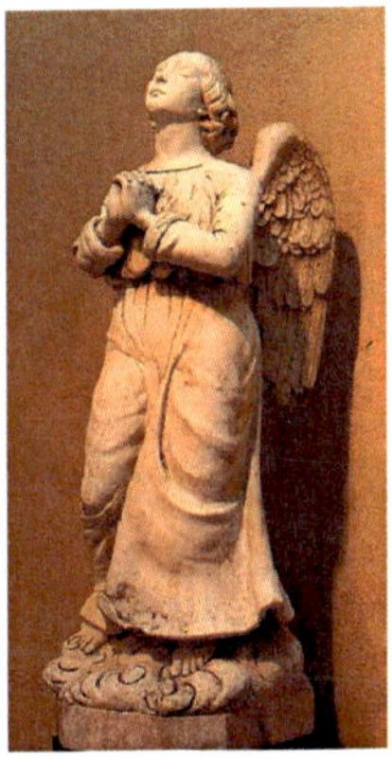

Priceless heirloom.

A collection of miscellaneous small articles for sentimental, decorative or other reasons is called bric-a-brac. The passage of time leads one to accumulate these items which have very specific value to the owner, evoking (hopefully) pleasant memories. So we try to display these things on shelves and in cabinets, to maintain a connection to the past. Something like: "Your grandma inherited this figurine of an angel, and it's been passed on for hundreds of years."

But what about the passage of a different kind of entity; a bric-a-brac of evil tidings: a BRCA1/BRCA2 mutation?

Both BRCA1 and BRCA2 are related proteins that can undergo harmful mutations which can dramatically increase the risk of developing breast, ovarian, fallopian tube, and prostate cancer. There may be an increased risk of other cancers as well. The proteins (of which I'll talk about BRCA1 as a representative) are present normally in what is called the wild-type gene, in all different kinds of normal cells in the body. BRCA1 is a normal constituent most of the time in humans, but for whatever reason, it is present in an abnormal mutated form in about 1-5% of all breast cancers, and although originally thought to be a genetic abnormality almost entirely confined to Jewish people of Eastern European extraction (Ashkanazi), this is no longer true; it's present in many different races. In fact there are at least 6,000

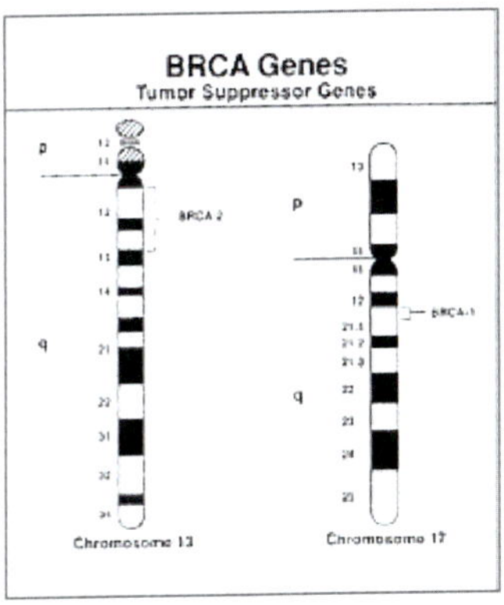

BRCA1 and BRCA2 are two genes associated with an increased risk of breast cancer: Many other genes of this type will be discovered.

mutations of the BRCA1 gene (11). Some of these mutations are of unknown significance in terms of the the precise function of the BRCA1 protein, which functions as a tumor suppressor gene in its native (wild-type) state. So in other words, BRCA1, when working in its normal state, prevents cancers from occurring by helping to repair damaged DNA (along with other functions). When abnormal, BRCA1-mutated breast cells are much more likely over time, sometimes after more than 50 years of waiting, to become invasive breast cancer.

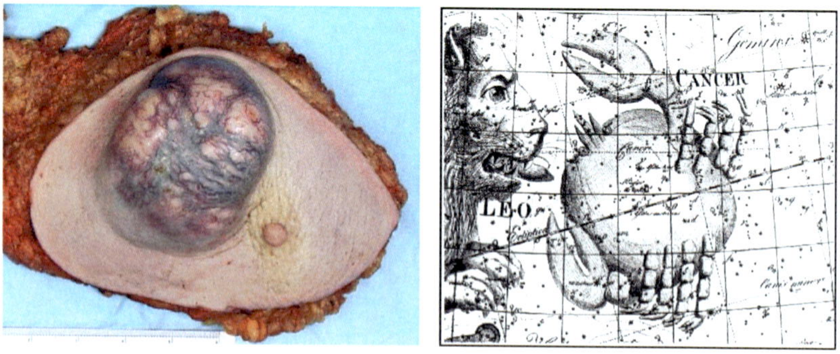

This is the terrible image of an advanced breast cancer and (with a very vivid imagination) its similarities to a crab (cancer in Latin) and constellation.

This is true for other cell types as well, for this mutated gene may be more critical in the development of breast cancer, but the gene is present in some fashion or form (active or inactive), in every cell in the body. And this includes the cells involved in creating people, in a process called gametogenesis, which leads to the production of abnormal sperm genes or egg genes (or worse, both), which leads to the potential transmission of BRCA1 to future bric-a-brac inheritors.

Now consider that it has taken us about 150 years to reach the point where we can talk about the inheritance of mutated breast cancer suppressor genes. And the first person to really understand the basic principles of genetic inheritance, had no idea what a gene was (the word was invented after his death, and rediscovery of his work), no idea what DNA was, no idea what a protein was, but he did know the difference between a tall pea plant and a short pea plant.

For God's work in creating all manner of thing includes the humble pea. He appeared to Moses as a Burning Bush, unconsumed by the flames, so His interest in plants is not a stretch. Nor is His sense of humility. For the man who discovered the fundamental laws of genetic inheritance was a lowly Augustinian monk, Gregor Mendel.* Yes, a priest was the one who over eight years of observation of simple breeding experiments with pea plants, after growing, recording, and analyzing data from 29,000 plant experiments, identified a pattern of transmission of something that led to reproducible predictions about the way genetic information flows.

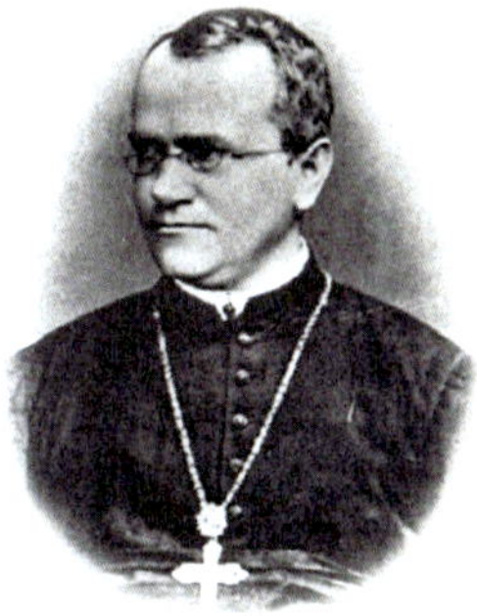

Gregor Mendel (1822 - 1884), priest and peaologist.

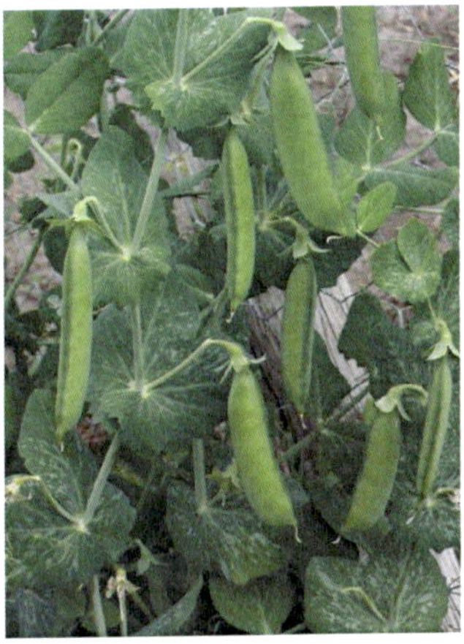

Pea genetics.

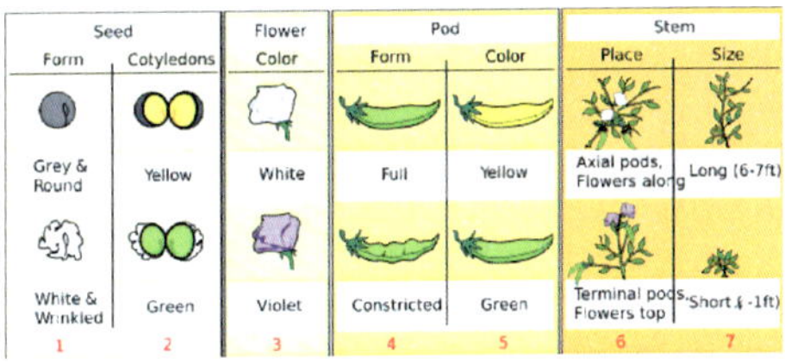

This great discovery, although ignored for more than 30 years, was eventually resurrected, after Mendel's death, and has become the essence of genetics. In fact you can look up the BRCA1 mutation and related information on the internet through the late Dr. Victor McKusick's website (Mendelian Inheritance in Man) http://www.ncbi.nlm.nih.gov/sites/entrez?db=omim which remains one of the great reference textbooks for all sorts of genetic disorders peculiar to our species.

The discovery of BRCA1, in 1990, by Dr. Mary King and her colleagues, was a great event in the history of genetics (12).

* Mendel remained lowly in the eyes of God, but did rise to the rank of Abbot of the monastery.

Yet it is particularly ironic that about 15 years before, she discovered that about 98.5% of human and chimpanzee DNA is essentially identical. Let us then be very humble and circumspect about from whence we came. Nor should we be too hasty about accepting all the claims of evolution, based on genetic identity, or any other theories that seek to explain how our species came into being. These are mysteries upon mysteries, "mysterium tremendum," which cloud our ability to understand where we are in the universe.

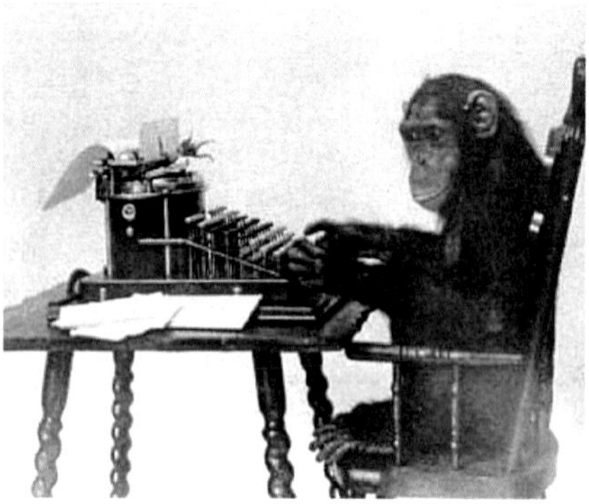

The author hard at work.

Rather than invoking the reductionist approach, consider that there is no fundamental contradiction between religion and science. It is only a reflection of our lack of true knowledge and understanding and insight into the impossible complexity of all things.

The Bible and other Holy writings from other religions are true within the Divine thought system that created them. My belief is that if God wanted everyone to be the same, to think the same, to do the same, then He would have made it so. But every objective and scientific observation I can imagine suggests that God, the Creator of the Universe, loves to be creative!

Now before you think that the Bible and evolution are in competition for our intellectual affection and devotion, think again, for they can both exist as independent thought systems, designed to be true within the framework of reference of the observer. It's no different than trying to measure time, and that may be why we say, "for a second to God is a thousand years to man."

So consider: Moses died. And Joshua died. But beyond the Biblical events, we are here to learn about cancer and science and medicine, and everything that encompasses that realm of human knowledge.

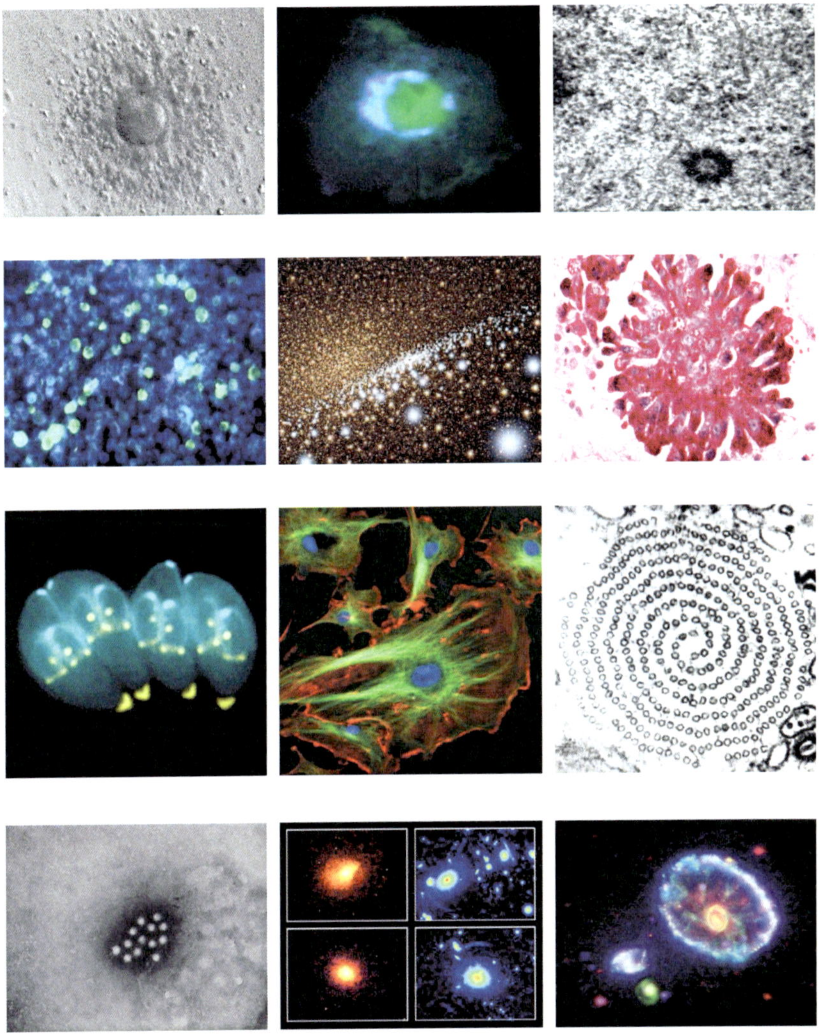

Cells, viruses, galaxies, stellar dust. Expressions of the Creator's absolute and perfect genius.

Moses Judah Folkman recently died. He helped put tumor antiangiogenesis inhibitors on the treatment map. With the use of Avastin, we are better able to control tumor growth by inhibiting blood vessel development that many cancers need to grow and spread.

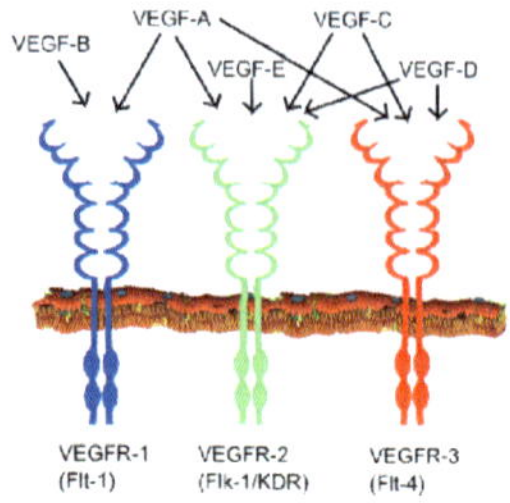

Avastin is a monoclonal antibody that binds to VEGF receptors and inhibits their function.

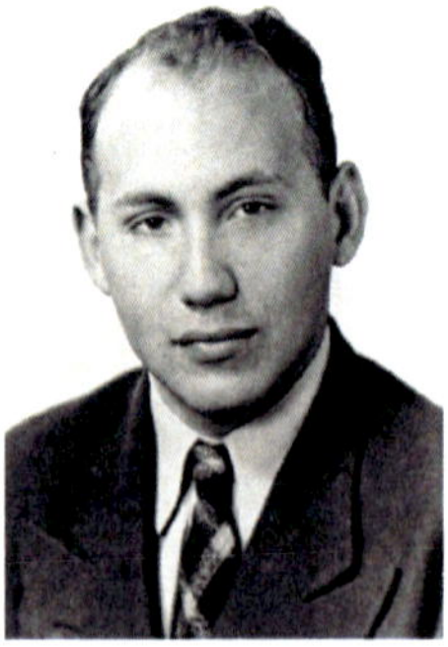

Dr. Lederberg in his 20's. He left medical school to pursue a Ph.D. in genetics.

Joshua Lederberg recently died. He discovered the role that sex plays in bacterial genetics. In understanding bacterial genetics, scientists were able to analyze the genetics of multicellular organisms, and eventually human genetics. So important was his discovery, that he won the Nobel Prize at age 33 (a very young age for a winner in Medicine) more than 50 years ago.

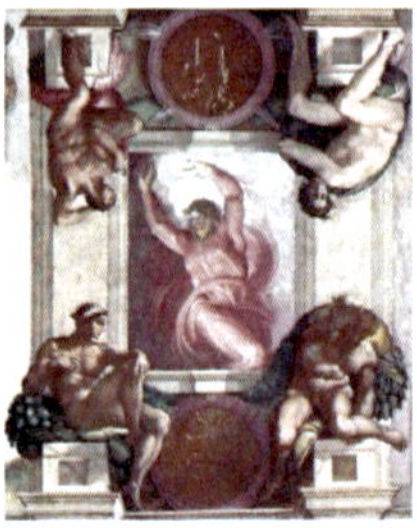

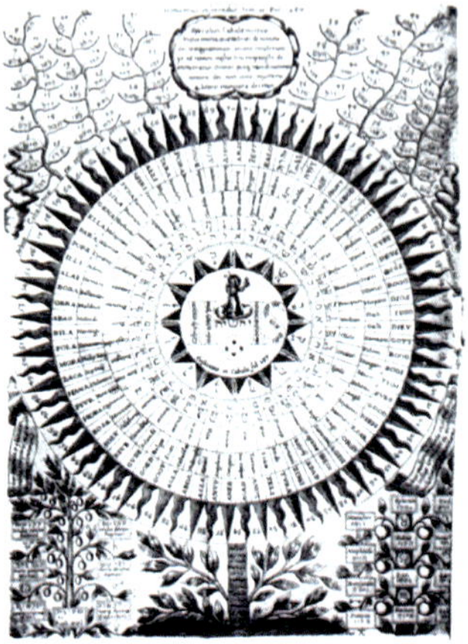

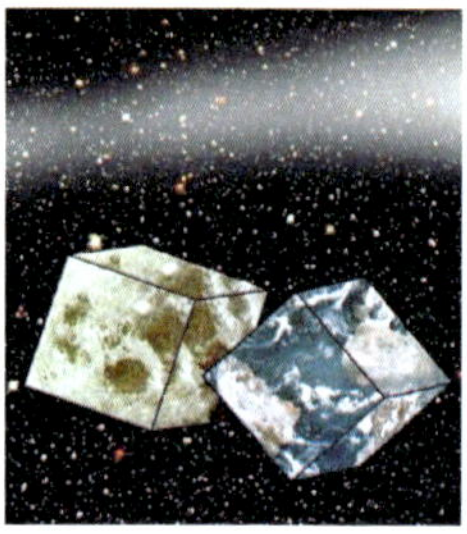

Mysterium Tremendum.

For we are nothing more than the dust of the Cosmos.

And Moses Judah Folkman and Joshua Lederberg were both Rabbi's sons.

IX. The Silence of the Worms

~~... if all the matter in the universe except the nematodes were swept away, our world would still be dimly recognizable.~~

Nathan A Cobb (1859-1932)

One function of these essays is to inform our readers of new and exciting developments in science and medicine that may be relevant to understanding and treating cancer and other diseases. So I am pleased to inform you about a meeting that took place in Brisbane, Australia, on July 13, 2008, which may have altered the course of human history.

The Society of Nematologists held its 5th International Congress!*

You can register online for the next meeting but space is limited, so hurry.

Why am I troubling you with making flight and hotel reservations, when you are busy trying to cure cancer?

So begins a story that is so incredible it must be true.

First, we must remember Rudolphi and celebrate the 200th anniversary of his discovery of nematode worms.

Next, we should praise tropical medicine doctors who throughout the ages have battled diseases with exotic and scary names like Dracunculiasis, Filariasis, Loa Loa, Ascariasis, and Trichinosis.

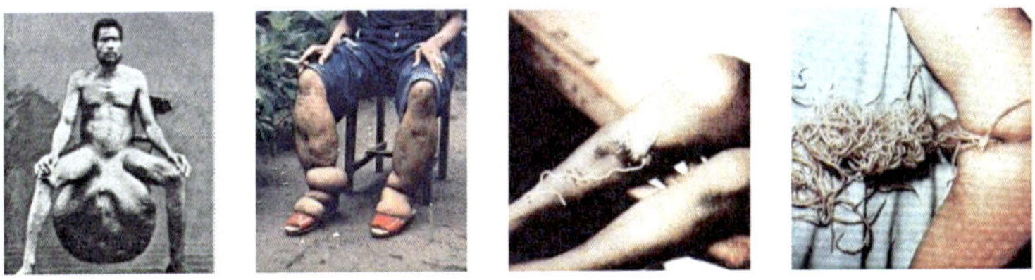

The terrible consequences of nematode infestations in humans. These images are not for the squeamish or faint of heart.

* **Sorry we missed this meeting. There will be others.**

In 2008, more than a billion people in the world were infected with various nematode parasites. As any medical student will tell you, the graphic images of patients with elephantiasis (where a limb or other body part can swell to incredibly disgusting proportions), caused by some of these parasites when they clog up lymphatic channels, make one aware of the terrible consequences of infection. And Onchocerciasis is a leading cause of preventable blindness in the world to this day.

Among more than 20,000 known species of nematode worms, many are helpful to mankind in that they eat bacteria and other things that cause disease in humans, and help regulate the life cycle of this planet.

But as my friend Nancy in New York would say, "Yeah, so."

Well how about two out of the last seven Nobel Prizes in Medicine?

For intrepid scientists more than 30 years ago, and in particular Dr. Sydney Brenner, one nematode stands above all others at 1 mm in length and at around 1,000 cells soaking wet. Whereas we humans are many trillions of cells in size and more than 1 mm hopefully.

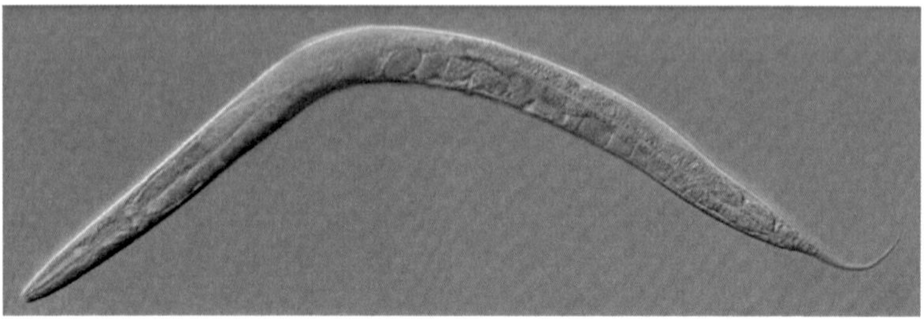

Superstar worm.

Its stage name is C. elegans; Caenorhabditis when its mother is mad at it.

Its claim to eternal scientific fame may rest on its diminutiveness, life cycle (7-10 days), and transparency. Not to ignore its capacity to survive frozen or (in a morbid sidebar) to survive even the Columbia spaceship disaster!

So when Dr. Brenner, Dr. John Sulston, and Dr. Robert Horvitz, were honored in Stockholm in 2002, C. elegans should have been at the podium too. And it wouldn't surprise me if they were real close, somewhere in the soil on the Nobel Foundation lawn, begging to get in.

By understanding the regulation of the life and death, and in a way the fate of each cell of this little naked worm, cancer may someday be treated with highly effective and novel drugs.

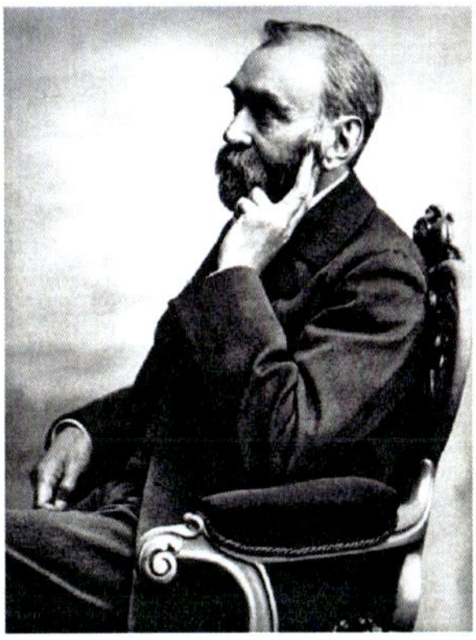

Alfred Nobel (1833-1896), inventor of TNT, and Founder of the Nobel Prize. Winners in each category receive about 1.5 million dollars (equally divided if it is shared).

In cloning the genome of this multicellular eukaryotic organism (the first), and in mapping the process of cell division and differentiation, and in understanding the genetics of this process, those scientists were properly honored. Because, their very important observations allow us to better understand how all living things function. For the same basic mechanisms that control life and death in this worm also work in a similar, but more complex, fashion in humans.

In further studies of this worm, yet another Nobel Prize was awarded to Dr. Andrew Fire and Dr. Craig Mello in 2006.

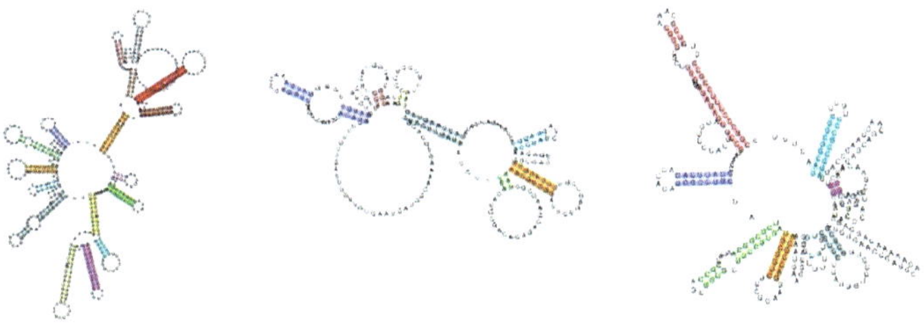

Three examples of different RNA forms of great complexity.

What these scientists discovered in C. elegans, that superstar of worms, is that genes could be interfered with by adding a specific mixture of RNA molecules, called double-stranded RNA. And in so doing, the products of these genes, proteins, could be prevented from being produced. And by "silencing" these genes, the function of cells could be dramatically altered.

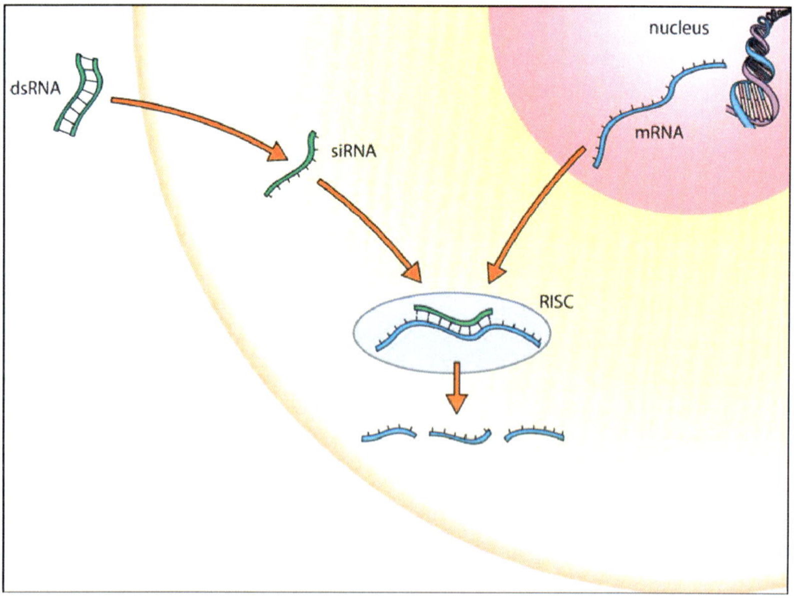

RNA interference was not discovered when I was in graduate school. It is yet another layer of cellular regulation and control.

Now biotech companies are studying various silencing RNA molecules in pre-clinical and clinical studies that could revolutionize the treatment of cancer. By shutting off specific genes that can promote the growth of cancer cells, using exquisitely specific molecules, one can hopefully avoid many of the complications that occur with conventional chemotherapy, which are directly related to the relative lack of specificity of these toxic drugs. (13, 14)

So when your children come back from playing in the nematode inhabited yard all muddy, compliment them on their spirit of scientific enquiry, and think, "Maybe someday a trip to Stockholm."

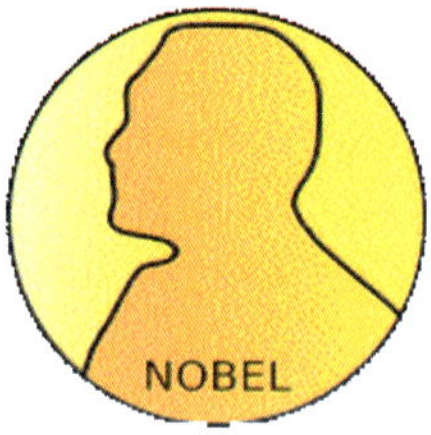

Maybe someday your muddy kid will win "The Prize."

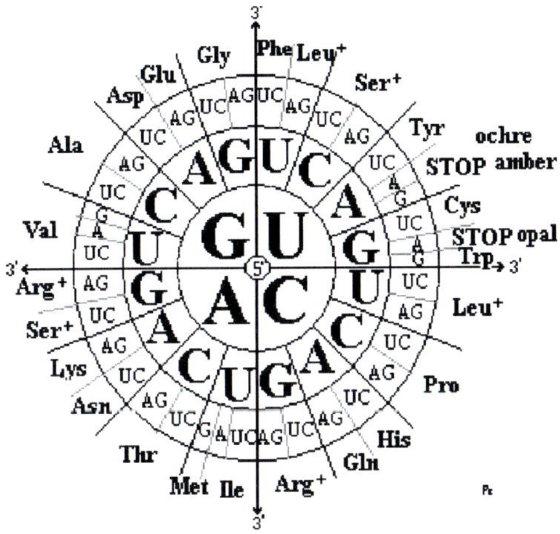

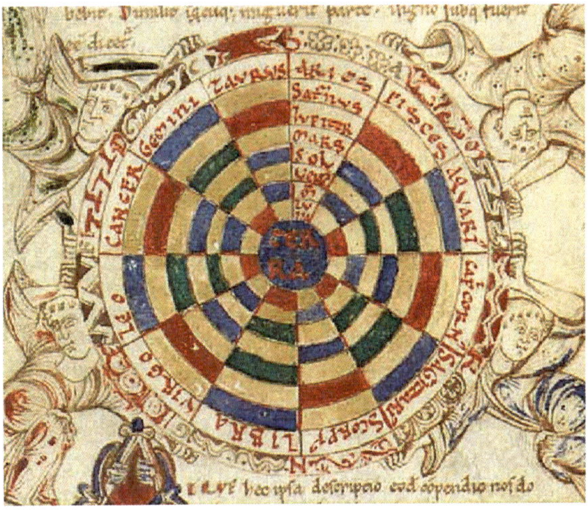

Convergence of forms: RNA code and a 12th Century view of the universe.

X. The Riddle of the Sphingolipid

~~It is, I think, particularly in periods of acknowledged crisis that scientists have turned to philosophical analysis as a device for unlocking the riddles of their field."~~ Thomas Kuhn, Ph.D. (1922-1996)

Years ago at a fellows meeting sponsored by a pharmaceutical company, I presented an abstract (which is a brief summary of work in progress), and spoke to the other attendees, in what was considered by many to be at best an adequate talk. But, it was much better than my performance in Rio de Janiero, about ten years before, when I stood before the audience, at the University of Rio de Janiero, and said nothing! I was absolutely terrified, and suffered from stage fright, which totally incapacitated me, so completely, that I could not utter a single word. My embarrassment was only magnified, for while visiting Brazil, I was the guest of my friend and teacher, the great scholar and man, Dr. Luiz R. Travassos.

So there was a certain measure of satisfaction in being able to speak coherently: if not quite the Thespian, at least I didn't make a complete fool of myself, as I had done before. And as the topics are connected, separated by more than ten years, it gives me a sense of perspective on how we mature through events that at the time seem cruel and unbearable, and yet we survive, and sometimes benefit from them, in unexpected ways.

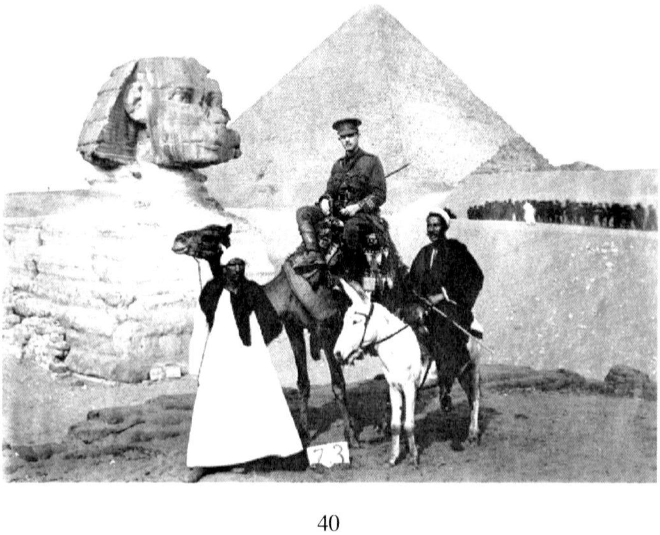

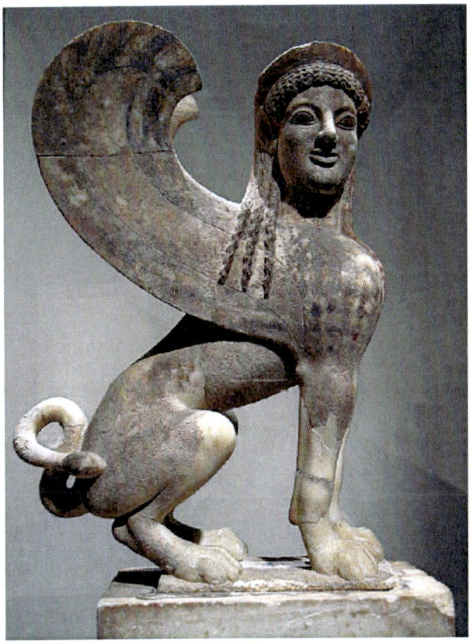 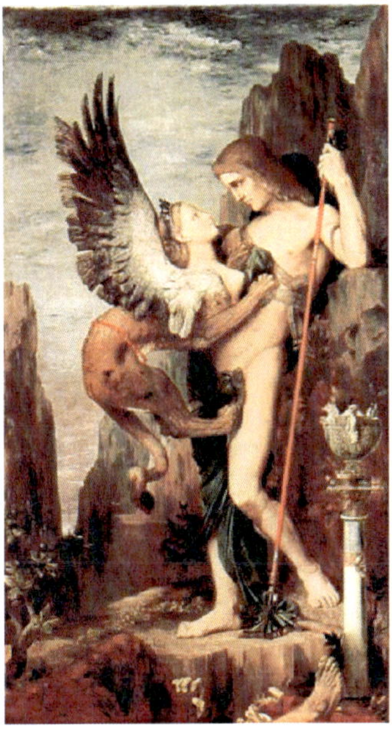

Solve the riddle or else!

As you probably know, the riddle of the sphinx was three questions. But before we get to that ancient story, and the origins of the Sphinx, let me tell you about sphingolipids which are not nearly as well known.

When we think about the basic constituents of a cell in let's say 5th grade, our teacher describes various structures or organelles. There is the nucleus, where DNA resides. There is the nucleolus, where RNA resides. We see images of centrioles, mitochondria, endoplasmic reticulum, Golgi apparatus, lysosomes, and so on.

But my personal favorite has always been the cell membrane. For a number of reasons, I love the cell surface. As in "I spent about ten years of my life, on and off, studying cancer cell surfaces." In simple terms, we think of the cell as a unique, biological entity because it exists to some degree, separate from its surrounding environment, yet, to some degree communicating with its surrounding environment through the cell membrane. The cell membrane is a double-layered lipid sandwich which contains many different types of lipids (cholesterol, phospholipids, sphingolipids, glycosphingolipids, and gangliosides* to name a few classes of molecules), which kind of float around as a sort of oily sea**, with many other types of molecules, interspersed as well, in what is a constantly changing environment.

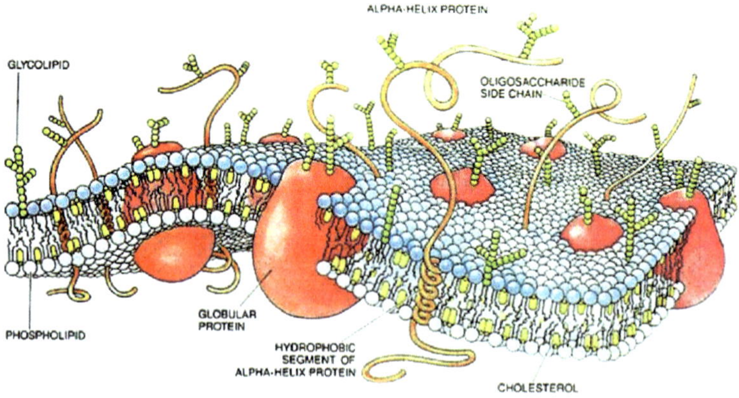

Cross-section of a small piece of the cell membrane and associated structures.

The cell surface, and specifically the outer part of the cell membrane, is that specialized part of the cell membrane that interacts with the external environment. Things are of course much more complicated, as sometimes parts of the cell membrane reverse sides, or flip-flop, and new additions are added, while other parts are discarded; and quite often, a layer of secretions from these cells, called the glycocalyx, accumulates just outside of the outer membrane as a sort of fuzzy matrix, which influences communication between cells and their environment.

So, now let us perform a thought experiment. I want you to close your eyes and think of the cell surface as a beautiful forest, with all sorts of amazing plants, and trees, flowers, shrubs, and grass, all dancing in front of your eyes, in a kind of molecular kaleidoscope.

*** More about gangliosides in essay XI "Lewis Thomas' Shoes"**

****Just before printing BP (British Petroleum) created an oily sea evolving in the Gulf Coast. This is a disaster of unspeakable magnitude.**

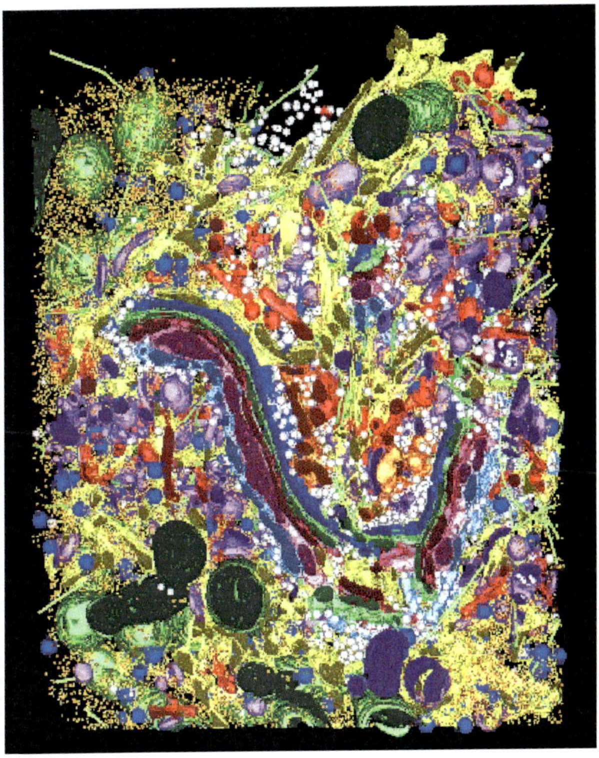

The cell as surrealistic art form.

To add to this imagery, now imagine a trillion cells, all with their own cell surfaces, with their own unique landscape. Now add the motion of membrane motion, to the motion of cells, to the motion of structures (organs), to the motion of organisms (us), to the motion of everything.

Whirling around, seeking out others, searching, probing, reaching out, constantly, wanting to touch, to embrace.

If you think of it as a way of achieving communion between living things, or as a subatomic spirit dance, maybe that will help.

Or maybe just another manifestation of the ineffable will and creativity of God.

Sphingolipids are molecules named after the Sphinx. The Sphinx was a god of Egypt, whose gigantic figure near the pyramids at Giza shows a human head attached to a lion's body. There are other sphinx permutations throughout Egypt, and over time the Sphinx became a Greek god, who assumed the form of a woman with a lion's body. Sometimes wings and a tail were also added. But, this was no lady! For she was quite fond of eating the unlucky people who failed to correctly answer her questions, with death and destruction her calling card, until her fateful end.

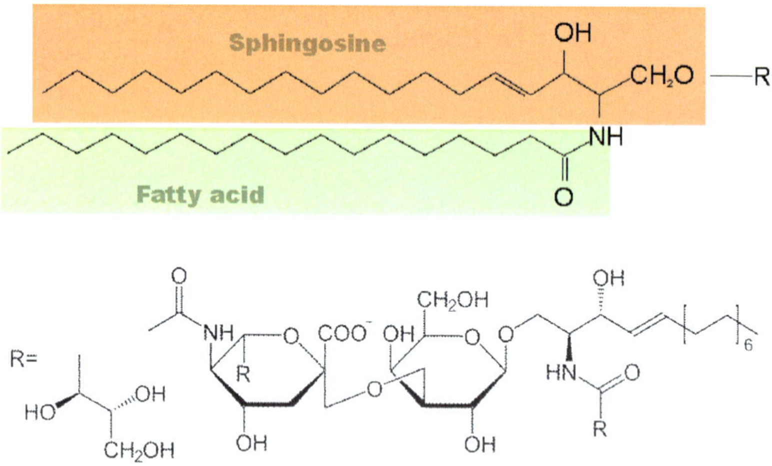

The two basic components of a glycosphingolipid: Sphingolipid embedded in the cell membrane with its polar carbohydrates sticking out to allow for cellular communication.

If I'd known the nasty behavior of the Sphinx when I was young, I might have reconsidered my choice of molecules to study. But the sphingolipid was cleverly named because it is in a way, the construction or joining of two distinct forms. A lipid portion typically contains a long chain fatty acid kind of like butter, and another part called sphingosine, both of which are connected and embedded in the lipid portion of the cell membrane. The other part, the "head", which sticks out into the cellular milieu, can be many different things. For instance, ceramide is a simple sphingolipid which ladies can find advertised in beauty creams. Sphingomyelin is another fairly simple molecule which allows nerve cells to conduct electrical impulses efficiently. A common disease, multiple sclerosis is an autoimmune disease that causes neurological dysfunction because of (in part), the destruction of sphingomyelin. The newest cosmetic phenomenon, Botox, a purified toxin derived from a poisonous bacteria, actually binds to (among other things), a class of sphingolipids called sialyated glycosphingolipids, which are also present on cancer cells, which I studied in the lab for many years. Even blood group antigens, which we commonly call blood types A, B and O, are often glycosphingolipids, and they are so incredibly similar in structure (and yet recognized by the immune system), that their precise molecular differences were not determined until the late 1960's by my scientific mentor at Sloan-Kettering Institute, the great biochemist, Dr. Kenneth Lloyd.

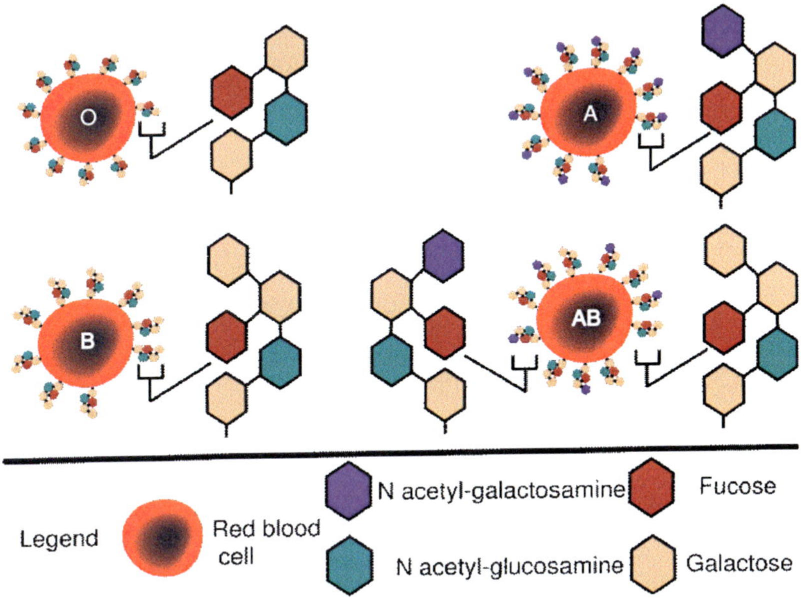

The human blood group antigen structure discovered by Dr. Kenneth Lloyd differ by the slightest molecular signature, and yet can evoke an incredible immune response if transfused to an incompatible person.

You must be wondering about the riddle, in the back of your mind, so here it is, as presented to the incredibly tragic Greek, Oedipus, who after his encounter with the Sphinx, through the whimsy of the gods, unknown to him at the time, killed his father and married his mother, then plucked out his eyes upon this terrible discovery and was killed by his sons. Which makes me wonder whether, in retrospect, answering the riddle correctly may have been the worst thing he ever did.

The riddle: Sphinx (licking her chops for it's suppertime): "Which creature in the morning goes on four feet, at noon on two, and in the evening upon three?"

Oedipus (feeling pretty good at this time): "The answer is man, who crawls as a baby, walks on two feet as an adult, and uses a cane in old age."

So the Sphinx destroyed herself, and Oedipus is perhaps best remembered by psychoanalysts who follow Freud's theory of an Oedipus complex in young boys, who reject and hate their fathers and love their mothers (which typically ends when they ask dad for the car keys and money to go out on a date).

Now the thing about the Greeks, is they loved a story with a message that overwhelmed the audience with emotion. Forget about my story doing that, but I can tell you sphingolipids, with ever so slight changes in their structure, location, or number, can lead to cellular destruction, or life. Ubiquitously present in the lowliest creatures and the most perfect (or imperfect) Greek hero, their structure and functions may be part of the solution to solving the riddle of cancer. So that with further study (thousands of papers having already been published), this story may ultimately end in a beautiful and joyful way.

XI. Lewis Thomas' Shoes

~~ Worrying is the most natural and spontaneous of all human functions. It is time to acknowledge this, perhaps even to learn to do it better.~~

Lewis Thomas, M.D. (1913-1993)

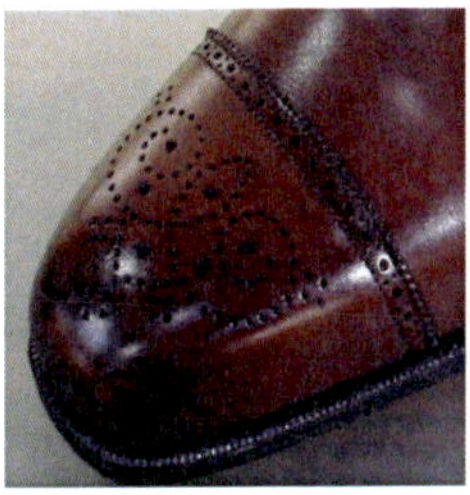

Wingtip shoe design. Both the author's and Dr. Thomas' shoe of choice (black preferred).

About 30 years ago I was on my way to curing cancer and in so doing winning a couple of Nobel prizes, and achieving world fame, I was also writing the great first novel, which would provide immediate recognition and wealth, while I accomplished more lofty goals related to ending disease, poverty, social injustice, war, and I forget what the other thing was.

Like Einstein, only with better hair.

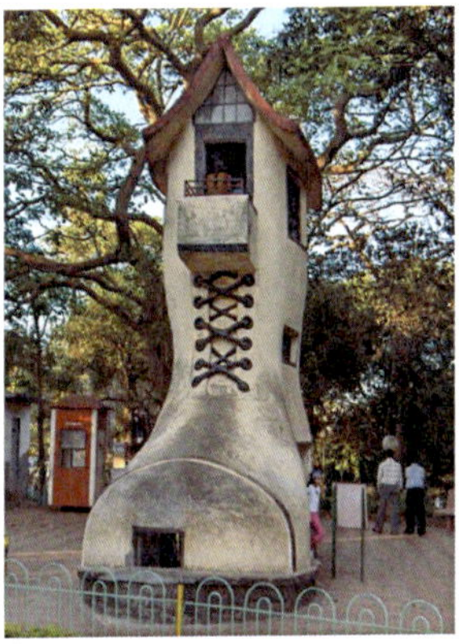

This shoe is larger than many NYC apartments.

It was a great time to be somewhat overly optimistic about my inherent abilities, for I think delusions of grandeur should be the province of youthful dreams to make the world a better place.

Part of that educational process included the great man's dress-for-success wardrobe. Fortunately, one day while walking to the lab, ready to tease out another mystery of creation, I caught a glimpse of Dr. Lewis Thomas, who at the time was Chancellor of Memorial Sloan-Kettering Cancer Center (MSKCC), in New York City. He was standing outside the Arnold and Marie Schwartz Research Building on 1st Ave and 68th St. and was getting ready to hail a cab. He was dressed in a conservative pinstripe suit and was wearing not just any shoes, but wingtip shoes!

Now I wear a conservative pinstripe suit and wing-tip shoes.

But the amazing thing is the coincidence does not end there. For Lewis Thomas and I are both MDs, both with lots of boxes of papers, both grew up in Queens, both had fathers who were MDs, although my dad was a "Meat Dealer" as the family joke goes, as in kosher butcher,* before he became a full-time cab driver. Dr. Thomas wrote beautiful books and I wrote....

Let's not spoil the story with a few details that are suspect. Instead consider that at Princeton University the Lewis Thomas Papers are housed, donated to his alma mater the year before his death, in 1993. This collection of stuff includes his expense accounts at MSKCC and totals 160 boxes, one of which is over-sized. I believe my wife and I are approaching that number. The reason I mention expense accounts is that I used an expense account... once.

The one time was when I traveled downtown to the meat district. I called the cab company (INTABORO) which I was working for (my dad let me drive his cab at night so that I could be a struggling artist of sorts), since for some reason my impressions of myself did not in any way reflect the world view at that moment in history. So while in Graduate School for a PhD in biochemistry (never completed), I drove a cab, and not too well at that. But imagine the sense of power and entitlement in calling said cab and being picked up for a round trip (with waiting time), all at the expense of MSKCC. Was I not special?

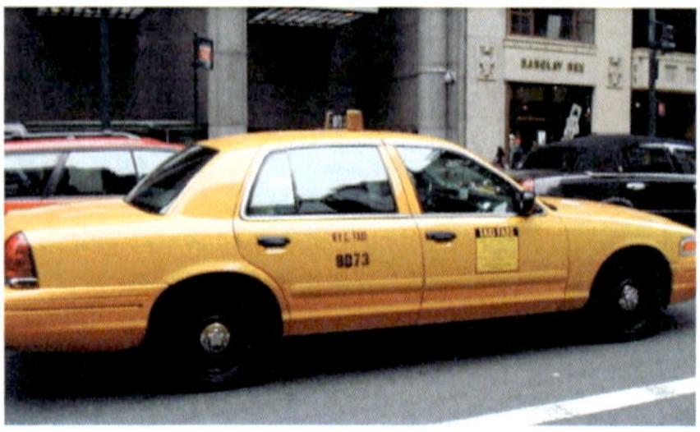

New York City cab similar to the one that both the author and Dr. Thomas rode in. Coincidence?

For this was a trip to Joseph Siege and Sons to obtain experimental materials which would change the course

*** My Grandpa Charley was a kosher butcher too and I loved visits to his store with vivid olfactory, gustatory, and visual memories still present nearly 50 years ago.**

of medical science. For Mr. Siege was selling me about one hundred cow eyes. Not to mention the chicken heads I had obtained at a nearby kosher butcher shop (no cab-- I walked), or the black molly fish obtained at a local pet store, nor the frogs my colleague Edward Natoli had shipped in from Long Island, which created quite a stir on the subway when they started to rouse from their cold induced slumber in the subway car, as Ed was not nearly as important as me* and so he had to take public transportation.

The end result of these zoological New York style safaris was that we were able to demonstrate that: 1) A monoclonal antibody (CR24) against a molecule called GD3 ganglioside reacted

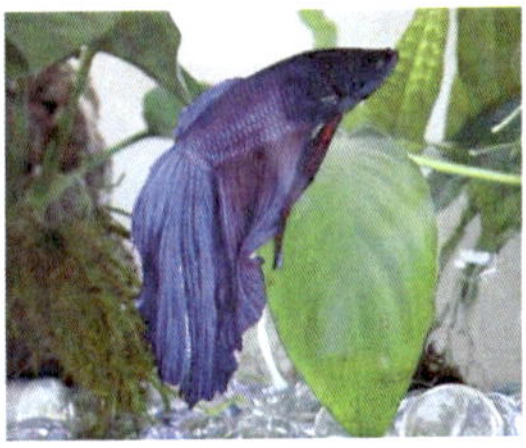
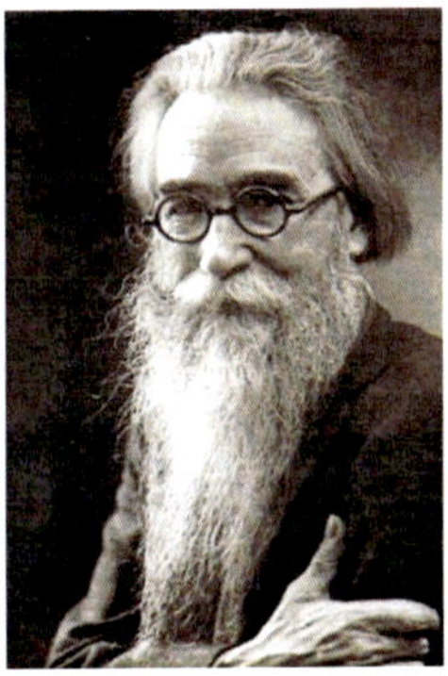
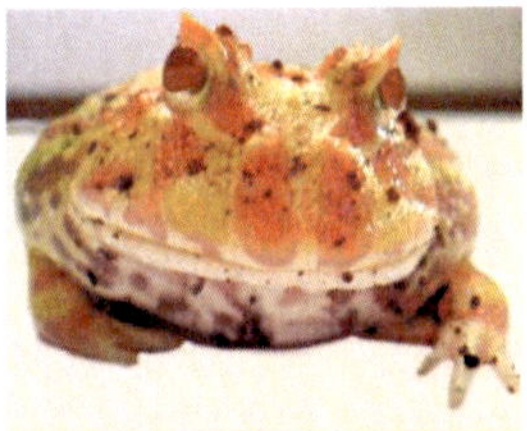

Fish, man, and frog all share GD3 ganglioside as a common molecule.

with melanoma cells and many other cell types, but it seemed to react with melanoma in a much more vigorous fashion. 2) Human antibodies from patients with melanoma could be sometimes detected that reacted to gangliosides on their own tumor cells, which we thought might be important in the way the immune system detects abnormal cancer cells and destroys them.

I believed that these observations were quite important in helping us develop methods to stimulate or promote the development of cancer immunity. As it turns out, things are much more complicated than just injecting a mouse monoclonal antibody to a tumor ganglioside and curing people, but the preliminary results achieved by Dr. Alan Houghton and his

*** My impression, not Ed's!**

colleagues while working in the lab of Dr. Lloyd Old, the great cancer immunologist, were incredibly encouraging. One of many problems was that over time humans make neutralizing antibodies to mouse antibodies, but to see people with metastatic melanoma sometimes have nearly all their cancer apparently disappear in a matter of weeks was fantastic. And in a special note of irony, I remember test review questions for the Medical Oncology boards, which were based at least in part on some of my earlier discoveries, I hope I answered them correctly.

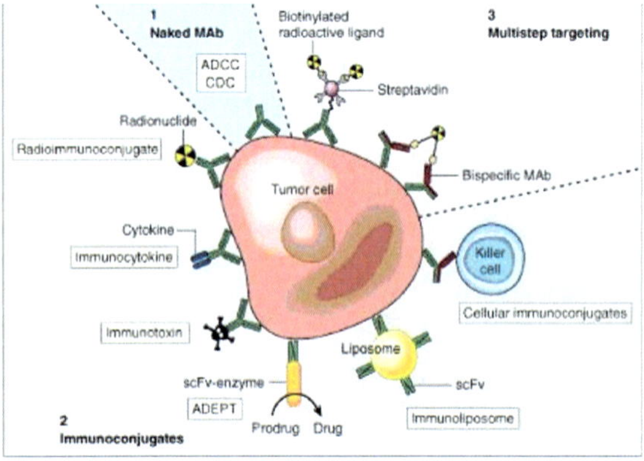

A carefully coordinated attack against tumor cells using very specific monoclonal antibodies is one of the most important strategies for the effective control of cancer.

Now the great Dr. Thomas had many beautiful ideas. His classic, Lives of a Cell: Notes of a Biology Watcher (1974), is one of several examples of his unique ability to synthesize profound ideas about science and medicine into a poetic form. And maybe someday when I grow up, someone will say something nice about my writings. But in the meantime let's tie things together in this essay, before you give up on me and run to purchase Dr. Thomas' books.

First, as far as I can tell, Dr. Thomas was many things to many people, and had an extraordinary academic pedigree. But his life's work was not entirely centered on understanding cancer. Nevertheless, he did suggest that the immune system was capable of detecting cancer cells and eliminating them through a process called immune surveillance. I suspect that one reason he is remotely remembered for this theory is his general popularity as a writer and scientist. But the fact is that other scientists were also thinking the same thing and were actively involved in the painstaking research needed to prove its correctness.

And like most ideas it was a long time in coming to the realization, despite a host of defeatists and naysayers, that it is fundamentally sound.

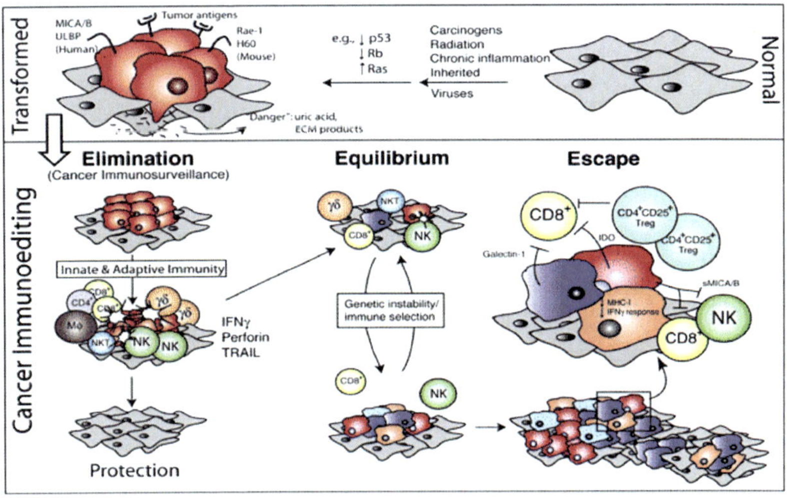

The three Es of cancer immunoediting: host protective versus tumor sculpting actions of immunity. Following cellular transformation and the failure of intrinsic tumor suppressor mechanisms, a developing tumor is detected by the immune system and its ultimate fate is determined by whether or not it is eliminated by the host protective actions of immunity (Elimination phase), maintained in a dormant or equilibrium state (Equilibrium phase) or escapes the extrinsic tumor suppressor actions of immunity by either becoming non-immunogenic or through the elaboration of immunosuppressive molecules and cells (Escape phase).

Dr. Schreiber, Dr. Old, and their colleagues have brilliantly described the way the immune system functions in controlling cancer. Sometimes incomplete success or failures do occur which leads to disease progression.

Which leads us "With a Wingtip and a Prayer" to the work of Dr. Robert Schreiber, Dr. Old, and many colleagues who have placed the immuno surveillance theory on solid scientific ground, an achievement for which they deserve the highest honors (15). In a process called immunoediting, (described in the figure above) the immune system, very often, detects and destroys cancer cells before they can become invasive and life-threatening malignancies. But not always is this system of control successful. What sometimes happens is that the cancer cells are able to escape immune recognition, in a manner of trickery and deceit, so the job now is to figure out how to help the immune system do better through the use of cancer vaccines and immunotherapy with humanized monoclonal antibodies and other methods of promoting a more robust and effective immune response to cancer.

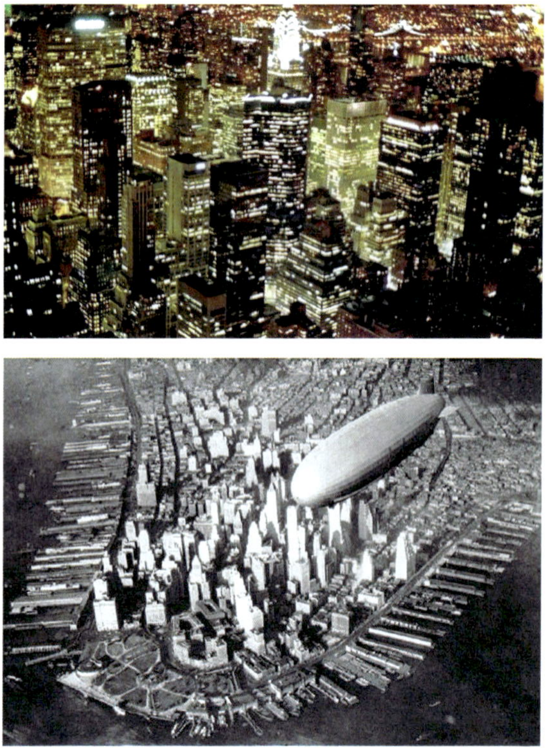

New York City: Images of a magical city.

XII. Can an Aspirin a Day Keep Cancer Away?

~~To do nothing is sometimes a good remedy.~~
Hippocrates (460BC-377BC)

Aspirin (acetylsalicylic acid) and similar substances have been known about for at least 2500 years! Hippocrates the great Greek physician (whose oath is still recited at medical school graduations) described the properties of a concoction derived from the bark of the willow tree which helped people with fevers and other medical conditions.

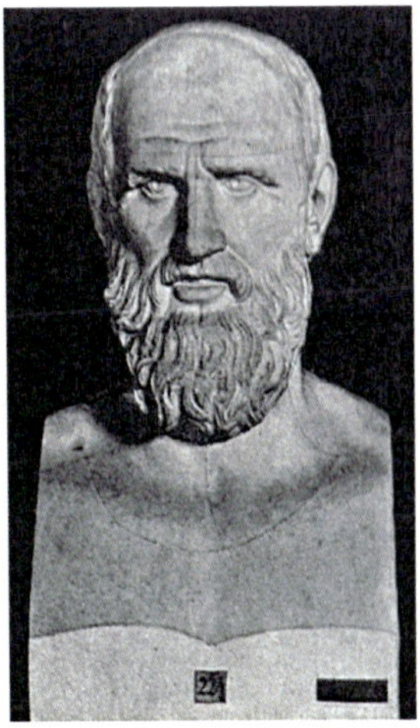

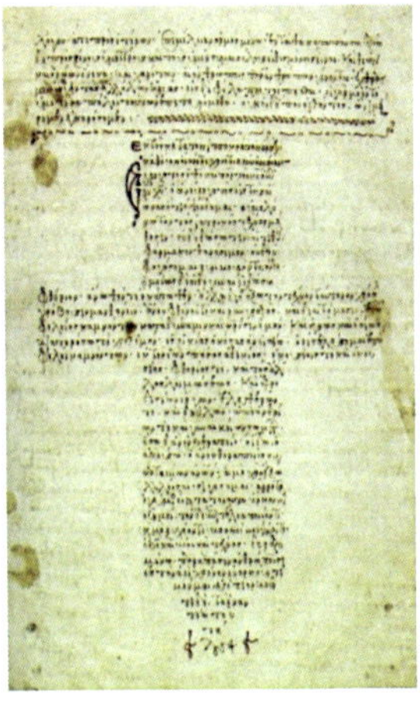

Hippocrates: The great Greek physician and his oath, "Above all, do no harm."

The Latin word for willow is salix, hence the name coined by scientists at the Bayer pharmaceutical company who synthesized this substance in 1899. And just in case you were thinking that anything from the bark of a tree is useless in treating cancer, I remind you that the chemotherapy drug Taxol was isolated from the bark of the Pacific yew tree.

Many scientific studies have been published which show that aspirin use can reduce the risk of various types of cancer. This effect is both dose-and time-dependent. The best-characterized example (16) showed that colorectal cancer risk is significantly decreased when people take aspirin about once a day (standard strength 325 mg).*

*** As this manuscript was in the final stages of preparation, "Hot Off the Press", a study by Holmes et al showed regular aspirin use decreases recurrence and death by breast cancer survivors. "J. Clin Oncol 2010; DOI: 10. 1200 JDCO.2009:22.7918"**

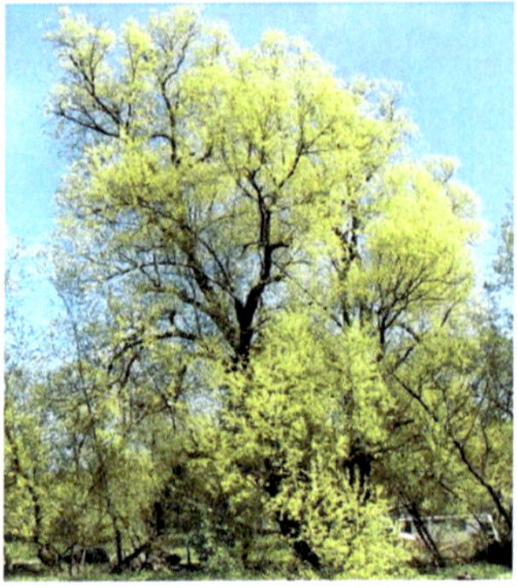

Willow tree: Original source of aspirin.

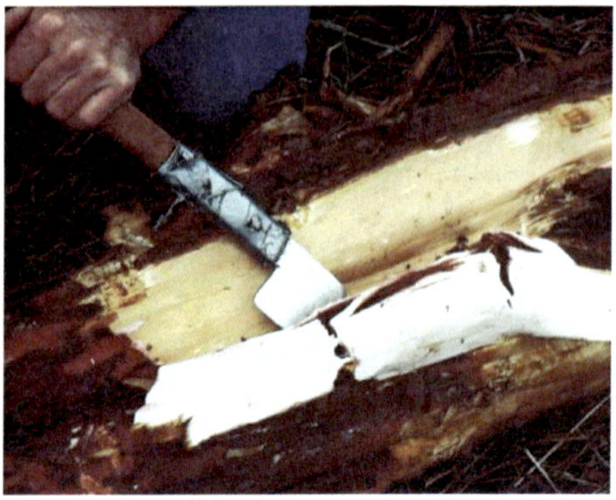

Yew tree Taxol "harvest."

Although the biochemical mechanisms are still being studied, we know that in tumors that over-express a specific enzyme, COX-2 (cyclooxygenase), aspirin use reduces the risk of colorectal cancer, but a clear statistical benefit is not observed in the population studied until about 5 years or more of regular use. About two-thirds of the tumors tested over-express COX-2, so that means in one third of people, the use of aspirin seems to have no benefit. This may also be true in other cancers such as stomach, esophagus, breast, and lung, although the data is not as mature or compelling yet.

More specific inhibitors of COX-2 have been in the marketplace for several years. Remember Vioxx? It is a COX-2 inhibitor that was withdrawn from the market due to an increased risk of heart attacks. Merck settled a class-action suit for nearly 5 billion dollars. But it, like Celebrex, may in some fashion be useful in treating various cancers, and there are studies that are continuing to answer that question.

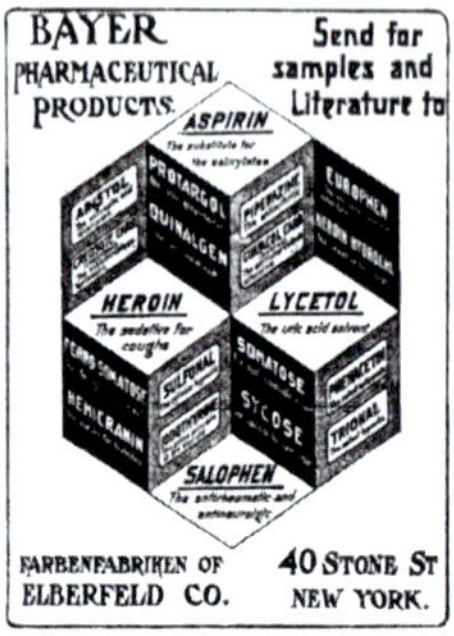

A reminder of earlier days. Bayer advertisement circa 1911. Heroin will be talked about in another essay.

It is entirely speculative, but I think that eventually tumors will be routinely screened for over expressions of COX-2. Inhibiting this enzyme and other enzymes,

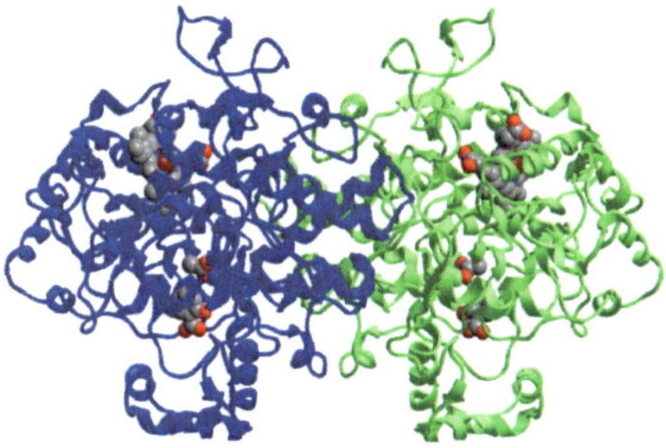

COX-2 enzyme inhibition by aspirin may help prevent cancer.

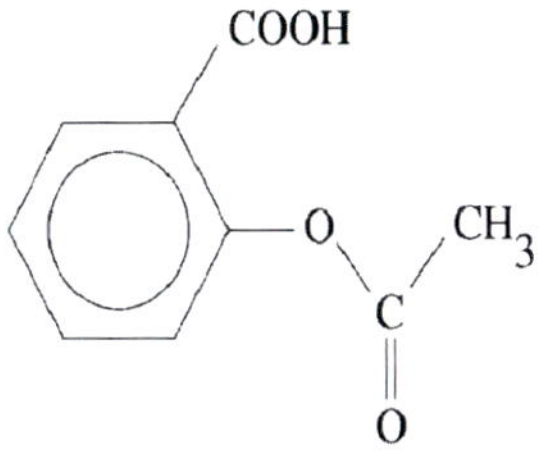

Aspirin structure.

with other biochemical pathway inhibitors, may allow us to treat various cancers with relatively nontoxic regimen. This might extend people's lives without making them so sick from conventional treatment.* I suspect that one of the reasons aspirin is not studied more intensely is its cost to the consumer is next to nothing. Another reason is our current chemotherapy regimens often lower platelet counts and together with aspirin, the risk of serious bleeding complications is very real.

So with the typical caution applied to taking any medicine (when in doubt ask your doctor or pharmacist, and investigate things on your own if so motivated), an aspirin a day may truly keep cancer away!

*** I looked up references to publications on "Cox2 inhibitors in cancer treatment" by entering the National Library of Medicine website PubMed. It's free for one and all. There were more than 1,600 studies! Many of these studies involved Cox2 inhibitors in combination with other drugs in treating cancer. There were also studies in patients with a wasting disease called cachexia that suggests Cox2 inbitiros as well. So who knows? Maybe I'll be right.**

XIII. Confessions of a Poppy Seed Bagel Eater

~~Thought: Why does man kill? He kills for food. And not only food: frequently there must be a beverage.~~ Woody Allen (1935-)

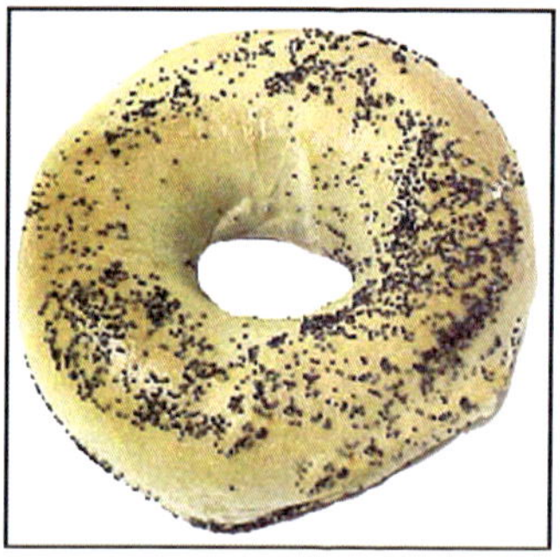

Poppy bagel: Caution! Controlled substance.

I'll admit it. I love poppy seed bagels with cream cheese and lox. Growing up in New York City, I never imagined that later in life as an oncologist, with a DEA license to prescribe narcotics and other controlled substances, I could theoretically lose my license to practice medicine by indulging in a culinary activity. To further complicate matters I also love poppy seed rolls, fresh from the same bakery pushers. So how can Mayor Bloomberg allow these acts to continue? But before you start to wonder about whether I really am impaired from the use of mind-altering substances, allow me to explain.

Let us then begin with the Papaver flower and its seeds. Imagine a neolithic cave 8,000 years ago. And in the cave is Ug the caveman. And he is really happy. For he has just eaten a bunch of poppy flowers and is feeling so good he's drawing pictures of deer and wooly mammoths on the walls, and there being no art critics, he is indeed pleased with his creative impulses. And then the former inhabitant of

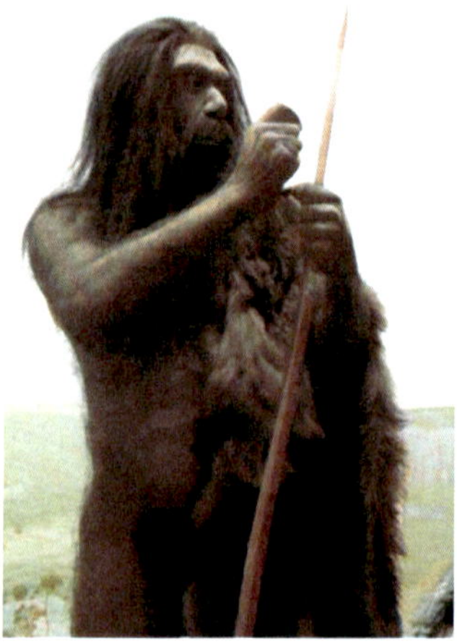

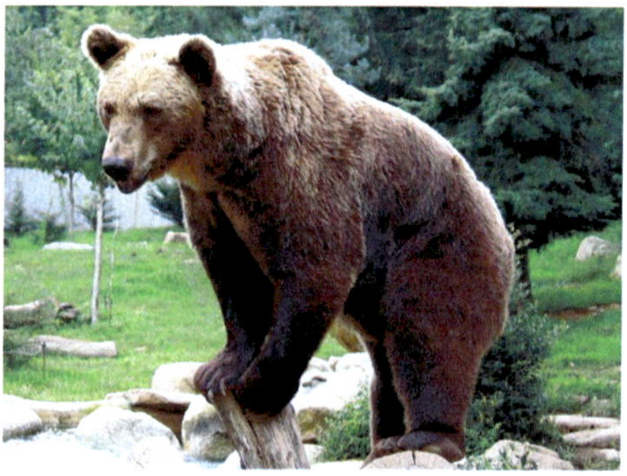

Ug and bear. Notice the bear is smiling.

the cave, a gigantic bear, comes back from looking for food and discovers Ug laughing and hooting it up. So now Ug is a poppy-induced fatality in the chain of life.*

Archaeologists discover the cave and analyze its contents and, being thorough, they find poppy seeds littering the place and there you have it.

But why trouble you with ancient history?

Well how about a sarcastic New Yorker who is addicted to cocaine and morphine? What can he teach us about history?

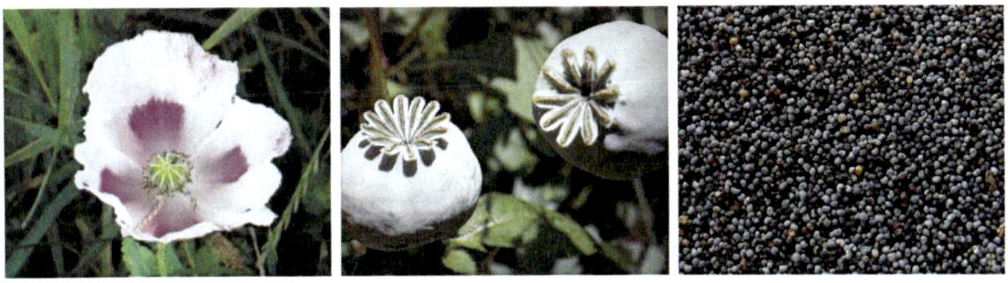

Opim flower, opium pods, poppy seeds: God's own medicine.

For starters, people have never forgotten the poppy, which is ironic because forgetting is one of the most reproducible effects of using narcotics derived from poppy plants. These narcotics are wonderful at stimulating brain receptors called opioid receptors and controlling the sensation of pain and they are also helpful in promoting sleep and a restful state, when used appropriately. The naturally occurring plant alkaloids derived from poppy plants are miraculous in their benefits to man and have been used by physicians for thousands of years. Opium contains morphine and codeine, for example, and there's the problem, for if you eat two poppy seed-embedded bagels or rolls and then are tested for drugs, you could be doing a lot of explaining to the authorities when you test positive for narcotics!

* The tragedy of drug abuse haunts us today and I offer no suggestions on how to reduce its destructive effects. A college student just recently died drinking tea made from poppy seeds and pods. (Newsrecord.org Tuesday, Oct 27, 2009)

Of course we're not talking about heroin, but we could be. For heroin is just another morphine derivative. It was created by Bayer chemists (yes Bayer, as in aspirin) in the 1870's and used for a variety of purposes including as a cough suppressant for children. It was also believed to be non-addictive so morphine or opium addicts could take it to get off the other stuff.

But in oncology, in treating patients in pain and suffering from terrible disease, there is no better drug than morphine and related opioid derivatives which differ only slightly in structure and potency.

Fentanyl, oxycodone, OxyContin, codeine, heroin, and methadone are all structurally related to morphine.

So when the Greek god Morpheus blesses us with sleep and dreams, hence the derivation, we have Ug to thank.

The great physician Sir William Osler* said more than 100 years ago, morphine is "God's own medicine." And this I believe.

What about that rude, drug-addicted New Yorker I mentioned earlier?

His name was William Halsted, and he and Dr. Osler changed the course of 20th century medicine.

At Johns Hopkins Medical School, they introduced the first residency program new for physicians and emphasized clinical training along with research as the basis for teaching medical students.

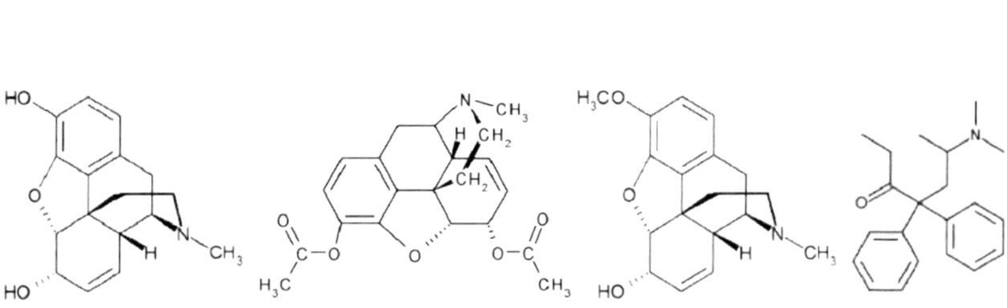

Morphine, heroin, codeine, and methadone: Most narcotics are structurally related.

* **More about Dr. Osler in essay XIV "The Resurrection of the Dread."**

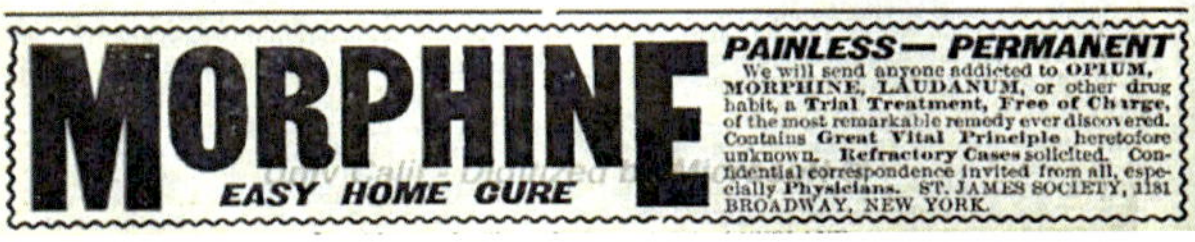

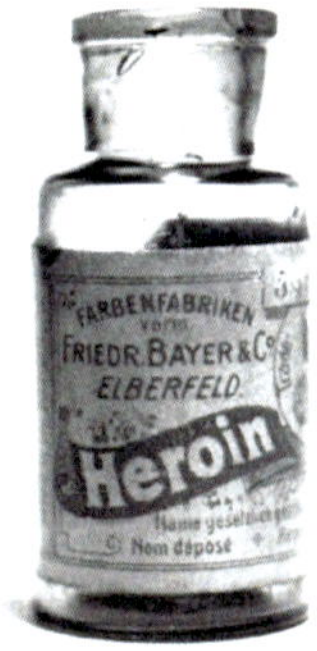

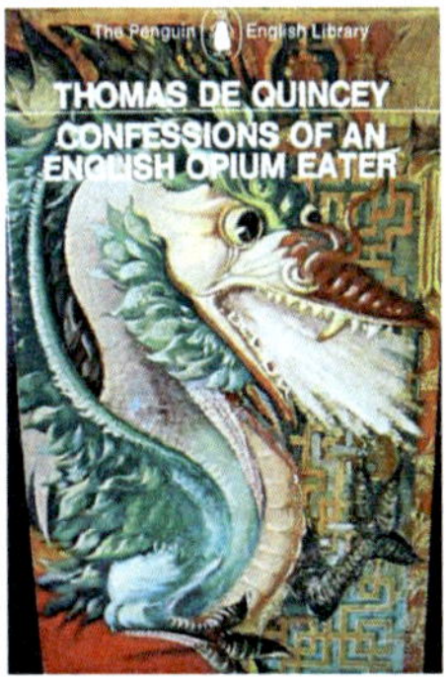

Early uses for narcotics in the days before the DEA.

Dr. Halsted was a surgical genius despite his use of narcotics and cocaine. He also smoked cigarettes like a chimney, and he could cut a surgical resident without a scalpel; a nasty word would do.

But as a Professor of Surgery at Johns Hopkins after spending his early career in New York, he trained some of the greatest surgeons in the world.

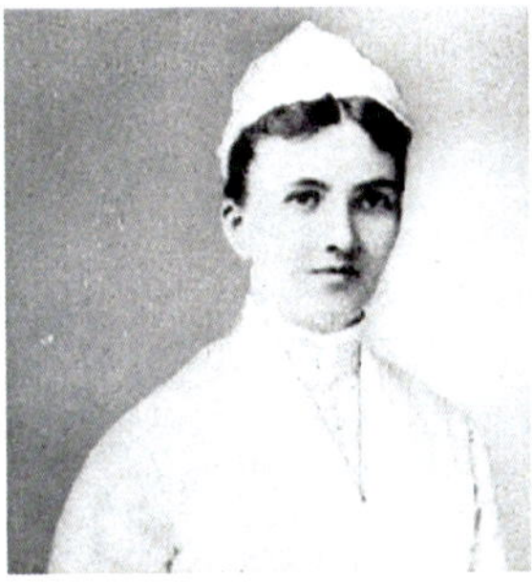

Mrs. William Halsted (Caroline Hampton)

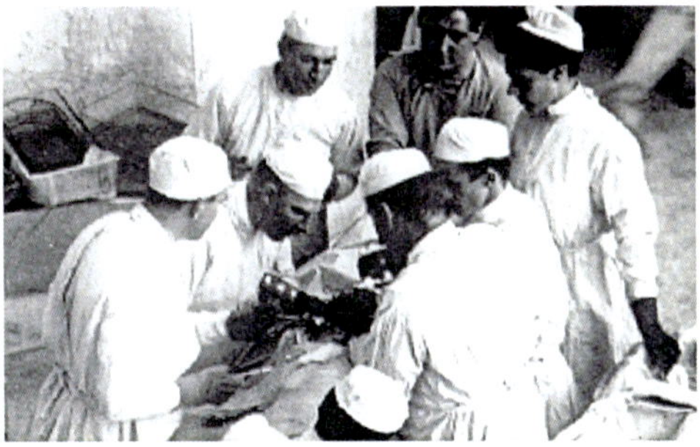

Dr. Halsted in Surgery.

Dr. and Mrs. Halsted helped change the course of modern surgical technique.

When his wife complained of sore hands from washing them in carbolic acid (she was his surgical nurse), he had the chemists at Goodyear Tire Co. create the first rubber surgical gloves. Before then surgeons would operate without gloves; he also realized that infection rates went down after their introduction, so that their use became the new standard of care.

But what does this have to do with cancer?

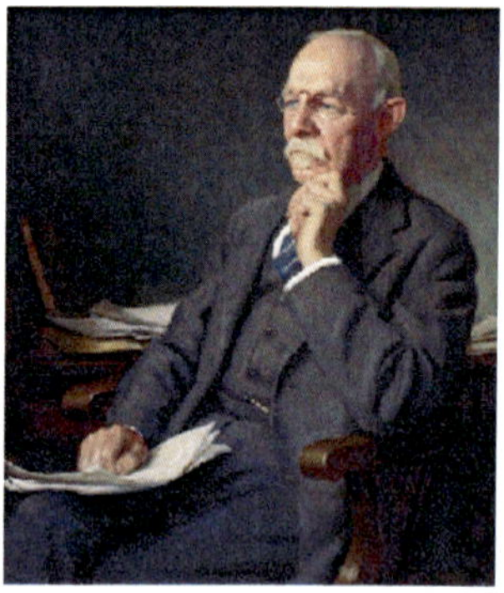

Despite the use of drugs, Dr. Halsted was a great surgeon.

Despite all the flaws of a Greek hero, Dr. Halsted cured women with advanced breast cancer with an operation that he invented called a radical mastectomy.*

This operation changed the course of cancer surgery and led to a less expensive modification of this procedure called a modified radical mastectomy where the chest wall muscles and some axillary lymph nodes are preserved. Even after more than 100 years, the basic procedure is the same, and as before this operation was invented there was little to offer women with breast cancer, his work stands out as a spectacular event in the annals of surgical oncology.

*** During the final editorial process, another "Hot Off the Press" item: For the Halsted aficionado, a must read *Genius on the Edge: The Bizarre Double Life of Dr. William Stewart Halsted*, by Gerald Imber, MD.**

XIV. The Resurrection of the Dread

~~First of all, let me assert my firm belief that the only thing we have to fear is fear itself - nameless, unreasoning, unjustified terror which paralyzes needed efforts to convert retreat into advance.~~

Franklin D. Roosevelt (1887-1945)

With a title like the "Resurrection of the Dread," I'll try to remain lighthearted as I write this. I want you to relax too.

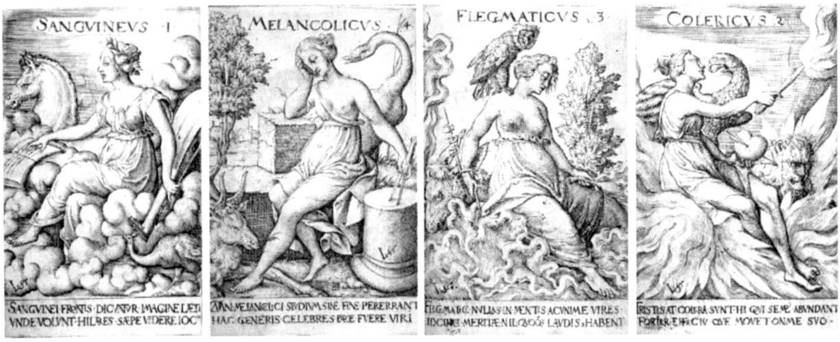

The four humors or temperaments (sanguine, melancholy, phlegmatic, choleric). A sanguine disposition is the most optimistic and pleasant.

Well maybe not lighthearted, but optimistic. Well maybe not optimistic, as much as fatalistic. On second thought don't relax.

Cheerful? Sanguine? Not really. How about hopeful? Yes, let's try to be hopeful!

So the title should read "Hopeful." Maybe, but when people come to see me with cancer for the first time, most often they are afraid. No, not afraid, something deeper, something closer to terror, but not quite, something like dread. So that's why I used the word "dread," as in "I dread seeing the oncologist next week, for what he may tell me."

Now what about "resurrection," as in a rising again or revival, and hence the play on words? For the phrase "resurrection of the dread" evokes a very primitive emotion in me (and I suspect you); it is a feeling inside us, of awe and great fear of the future.

So let's consider a real life example, of a case seen several years ago. A 60-year-old lady is admitted to the hospital when she comes into the emergency department over the weekend, complaining of severe neck pain, radiating to her head. On exam, an X-ray of her neck shows an area of bone in her cervical vertebrae which appears to be "eaten away," a so-called lytic lesion, suggesting some type of malignancy. She is examined by a physician who finds that her entire right breast (skin iincluded), is completely distorted, hard, and red and orange in color, along with hard, enlarged lymph nodes identified under her right axilla (armpit).

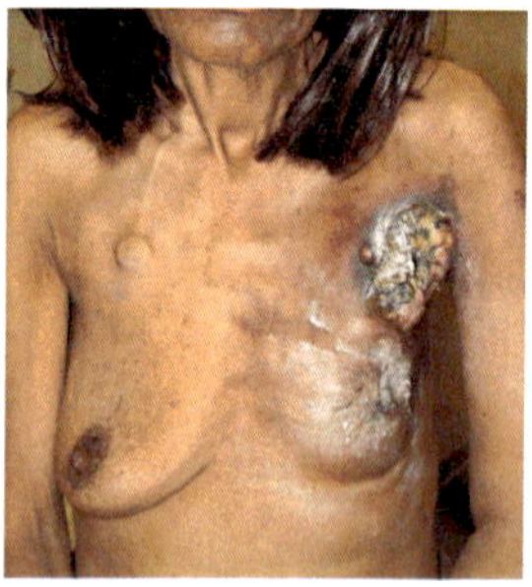

The destructive changes seen in advanced breast cancer, similar to the case described by the author.

In today's times, why believe in God? Why not believe in the incredible advances we have made in science, technology, medicine, and you name it, that our species, without Divine revelation, has conceived. Or better create a religion where there is no God: Atheism. Or just sit on the fence, and say "I'm not sure....the evidence....," or become God yourself (batteries not included). Or worship Satan, with the obligatory black on black on black wardrobe. Pascal's* wager is the best answer to alternative views about the nature of the Universe, in which if you believe in God, and He doesn't exist, no harm. But if you don't believe in God, and He exists, potentially big harm.

Personally, I really don't care what people believe in, as long as they leave me alone, and do not impose their beliefs on me. I feel the same way about my patients, most of whom have some measure of spiritual development which they can hopefully utilize to get through the difficult days ahead. If not, that's fine too; I can play the game any way you want me to. For it really is a game (the only game in town), where we bet that something we do will have a positive and salutary benefit. So we treat, and all the cancer seems to disappear, and we celebrate! Or we treat

*** Blaise Pascal (1623–1662) was a genius of the first order who was a mathematician, physicist and Catholic mystic.**

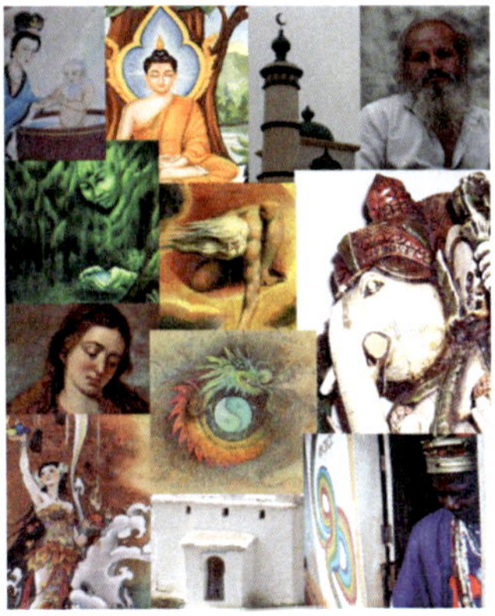

Who can begin to understand the ineffable will of God?

and the cancer laughs at the treatment and nothing we do works, and the patient dies soon after. Or we treat and it's a mixed picture where some of the cancer disappears, while other cancer stops growing for awhile. Or we treat and an extremely rare but fatal drug reaction occurs which actually causes death sooner than it would occur without treatment. You get the picture.

I don't know who will be around tomorrow let alone 6 months, or 2 years from now, nor will I ever know these things, nor do I desire to know these things, like some kind of perverse cancer handicapper, who in all seriousness, with neat and clean white coat, says: "You have only a short time left; I'm sorry."

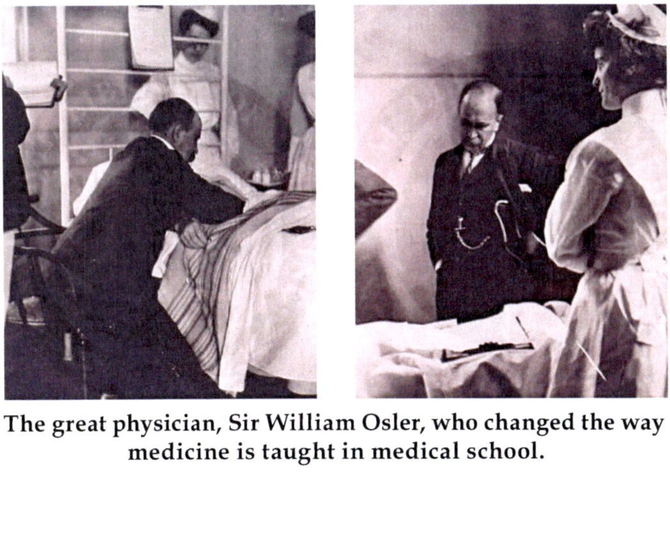

The great physician, Sir William Osler, who changed the way medicine is taught in medical school.

William Osler, MD, considered by many to be the founder of modern medicine, said it best (and I paraphrase): "One thing is certain. It is not for you (the physician) to don the black robe, and assuming the judicial function, take hope away from the patient, hope that is dear to us all." And from Cicero: "While there's life, there's hope." And from Samuel Johnson: "Hope is necessary in every condition." And from Aristotle: "Hope is a waking dream."

So why did this woman wait years before she sought treatment for breast cancer? I think the answer is that she was completely terrified, and hoped it would go away on its own, without treatment, just prayer. Which could have happened, but didn't. She dreaded the thought of cancer, so she ignored its obvious signs and symptoms, until her physical pain became unbearable. But her faith has prevailed and she's doing much better now on therapy, in both a medical (cancer shrinkage and much less pain), and spiritual way (as in hope for the future).

But what does "Resurrection of the Dread" mean in an oncology-specific sense? It is simply the human emotion (in an admittedly extreme form), of intense and somewhat irrational fear in seeing one's cancer doctor in followup!

In other words it is a rising up again or revival of all the emotions that one feels in life-threatening situations, such as a cancer diagnosis. So when a return visit is scheduled, very often patients are beside themselves, with great trepidation, about how they are doing. "Is the scan OK?" Translation: "Do I have to worry about the cancer returning and dying soon?" "I had a headache last week." Translation: "Am I dying from brain metastases?" "I have a spot on my arm." Translation: "Has the cancer spread to my skin?" And so forth.

Now this nice lady was not a primitive cave dweller. She is an otherwise healthy, sophisticated, intelligent, modern female who is a college graduate, living at a time in history when everyone is bombarded with cancer information. Yet, she waited a few years before she was forced to seek medical attention, not for her diseased breast, but because of excruciating neck pain from the breast cancer spreading to her bones and destroying parts of them.

As an oncologist who believes in personal freedom and the role of religion in the way people deal with disease, I saw the patient over the weekend, with her family present, and we talked about the likelihood this was metastatic breast cancer, while awaiting the breast biopsy results. I did not say: "You have breast cancer." I did not say: "How could you wait so long before you went to the doctor!" I did not say: "Your prognosis (translation in "Patientese": 'You're going to die soon') is poor."

I simply said: "As you already know, the likelihood is that you have advanced breast cancer, and the first things we need to do are be patient (waiting for the final pathology report), and start the so-called staging workup which would include a PET scan, and MRI, as well as laboratory tests, tumor markers, and such."

The other words said, before I left: "Courage, Patience, Faith, and Hope."

Nowhere was there negative thought, or speculation about the future. Despite some of my colleagues' insistence, we are not gods, nor can we prophesy. We are at best God's instruments. Or as the great 16th century surgeon Ambroise Pare said: "I treat the patient, but God heals the patient."

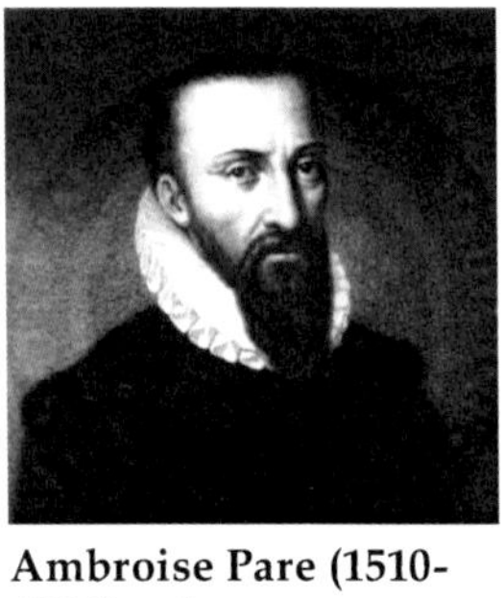

Ambroise Pare (1510-1590), who, among many innovations, helped develop modern surgical suturing and humane methods of wound healing.

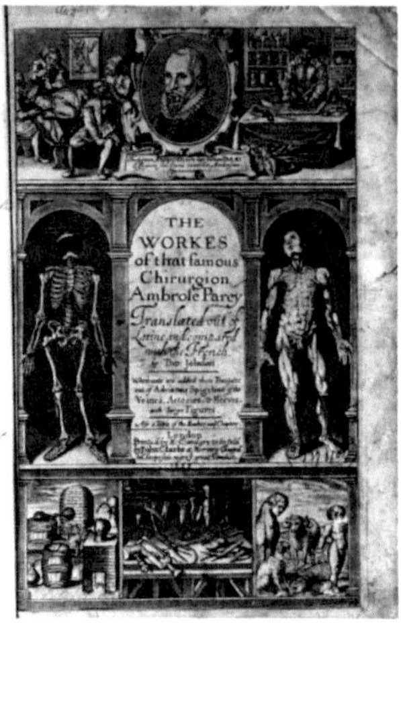

Let me tell you a secret: Whether anything works at all is a miracle! There are great miracles, small miracles, and everything in between, but I've been around too long to believe in anything else. I understand all the principles of medical science, have an excellent academic pedigree, treat people with the best available drugs based on the scientific evidence, but whether it works or not is not within my sphere of influence, that is the province of the Almighty. And as I've said many times to seriously ill people over many, many years of medical practice: "I know what I'm doing, and the Good Lord knows what He is doing, and He's running the show." "If He tells me what the outcome will be (many years of life or not), I'll let you know, otherwise, we'll just pray and do our best."

XV. Wilt Thou Indeed Destroy the Righteous with the Wicked?

~~Who is like unto thee, O Lord, among the gods? Who is like thee, glorious in holiness, fearful in praises, doing wonders?~~

Exodus 15:10-12

We begin with Genesis 18:23-33. Abraham meets God and they discuss the incredibly evil behavior of the people of Sodom and Gomorrah. God is planning to send his Angels to investigate further and dispense justice if needed. Abraham is afraid that God will destroy his nephew Lot and his family with all the others and so he begins an extraordinary dialogue with the Almighty.

Abraham: "Suppose there are fifty righteous within the citv. Wilt thou indeed destrov the righteous with the wicked?"

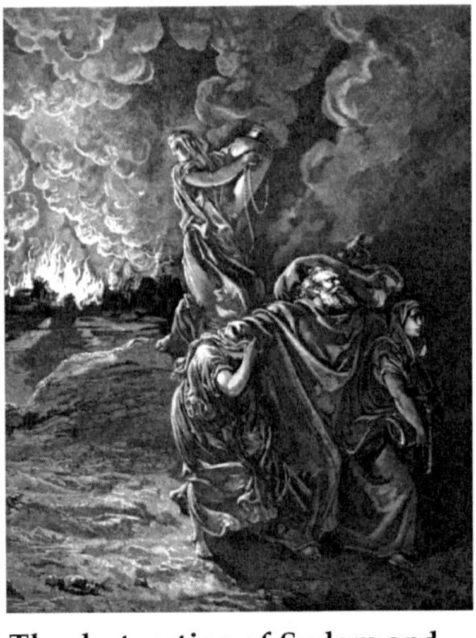

The destruction of Sodom and Gomorrah as Lot and his family flee. Notice his wife's curiosity got the better of her.

God: "For the sake of fifty I will not destroy it."

And so on until we get to ten, at which time God breaks off the negotiations.

God through his Angels saves Lot and his family, which was Abraham's primary concern, although the statement: "Shall not the Judge of all the world do right?" suggests more lofty concerns. Lot's wife does not listen (after they escape) to the Angelic instructions and so she becomes a pillar of salt. But Lot and his daughters live and after a terrible misunderstanding (his daughters thought they were the only survivors in the world), they co-habit and create a race of people called the Moabites.*

*** After their incestuous coupling, one daughter's child became the progenitor of the Moabites; the other daughter, the Ammonites.**

So a story about potentially unfair and indiscriminate treatment of innocent people ends in a way that only God could imagine.

A fair question is what is the relevance of this story in a cancer essay? But, and this is not a stretch, we often treat cancer patients in an unfair and indiscriminate way with incredibly toxic poison. The end result, (as the title of this essay suggests) although not as final and dramatic, is reminiscent of this ancient debate between God and man.

One could choose many different tumor types, but let's start with the statement that most often the treatment of breast cancer with chemotherapy drugs is ineffective, costly, and dangerous. The reason we accept this measure of treatment failure is because we have convinced ourselves that we are justified in treating everyone to benefit around 5 to 20% of patients. We have also convinced ourselves that if perhaps one or two people die from chemotherapy-related complications (per thousand), this is statistically acceptable (unless of course, I suspect, that person is you or someone you love). And let's add in about 20 people per thousand who develop irreversible health problems like heart failure or blood diseases, and maybe 20 per thousand with serious complications that are reversible but were potentially serious and life threatening like infections, allergic reactions and such.

So let's crunch some numbers. Treatment X: For every 1,000 patients treated at a cost of around 50,000 dollars per patient, 100 are helped in that they are cured of their disease (10%), one or two die from therapy, who may have done well without it, and 20 people are sick the rest of their lives, who may or may not have benefited from treatment. Nor should we ignore many people who have persistent side effects from treatment which never entirely disappear.

Let's call the treatment AC for Adriamycin/Cytoxan for early-stage breast cancer. For believe it or not, after about 20 years of using this regimen as the gold-standard in breast cancer, an observation by Dennis Slamon, MD, PhD, one of the world's experts in treating breast cancer, made me shudder. His quote from the 30th Annual San Antonio Breast Cancer Symposium (12/13/07): "Given the known long-term cardiac and leukemogenic toxicities of anthracyclines and the lack of incremental benefit in the non-HER2 population, we can ask if there is any role for these agents at all."

Before we get to the HER2 status of patients and its significance, let's talk about the history behind Adriamycin (doxorubicin) and Cytoxan (cyclophosphamide).

Adriamycin is an anthracycline drug isolated from a strain of bacteria called Streptomyces. In other words, it is an antibiotic that the bacteria produces to kill other invading microorganisms, including competing species of bacteria and fungal organisms. Other examples of Streptomyces-derived drugs which have revolutionized the treatment of infectious disease are a pharmacopeia Who's Who: Nystatin, Amphotericin B, Erythromycin, Tetracycline, and Vancomycin. Adriamycin kills all sorts of cells (both microbial and human), and that includes cancer cells. It inserts itself (intercalates) into DNA, and leads to cells dying because they cannot repair the damage to their DNA. This effect is as true with normal cells such as bone marrow progenitor cells, as it is with breast cancer cells and in fact as we now know, it is much more effective at killing bone marrow cells than breast cancer cells.

Cytoxan (cyclophosphamide) and its derivatives have been around for nearly 200 years, in the form of chemicals called nitrogen mustards. Yes, the same nitrogen mustards (with slight structural changes), that were used in World War I to gas troops. What happened after exposure, beyond terrible lung and skin damage, was that doctors observed a decrease in the number of white blood cells in some exposed soldiers. They tried treating leukemia patients with these chemicals and eventually tested them on many different cancers, sometimes with encouraging results. So by trial and error, so-called "empiricism," Cytoxan continues to be used in treating many different cancers and blood diseases, typically in combination with other drugs. We even use it in treating autoimmune disease such as systemic lupus erythematosus, since it kills off immune system bone marrow cells that attack normal body components.

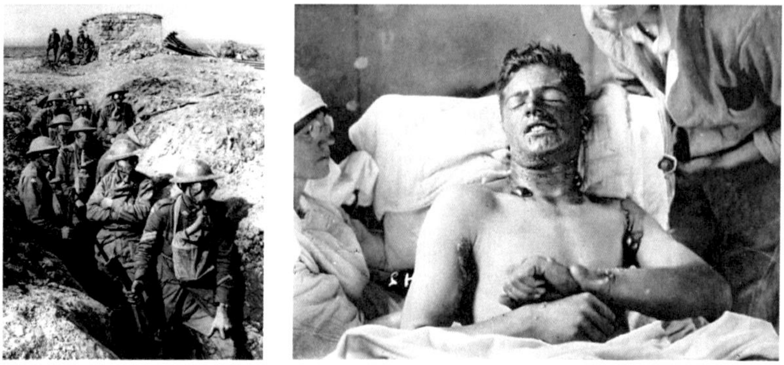

The origins of many chemotherapy drugs still in use are from "The War to End all Wars."

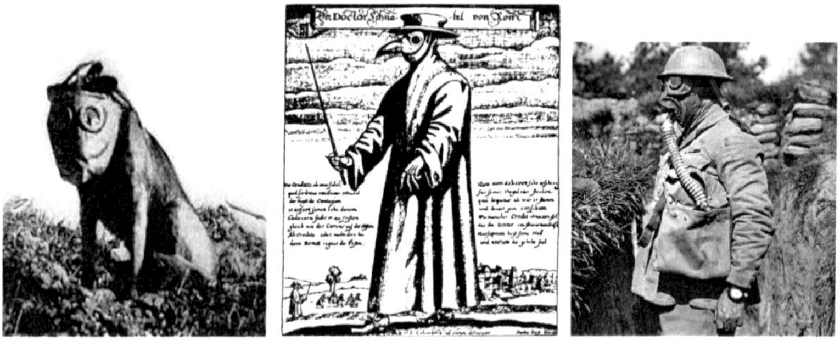

Dog, doctor, and soldier with masks to protect them from noxious vapors. The doctor's outfit is from the 17th century to protect against the black death and other epidemics.

So Adriamycin (named by Italian scientists after the Adriatic Sea)*, AKA doxorubicin (derivative of ruby red color), an antibiotic, is one of the most commonly used chemotherapy drugs in treating breast cancer and other malignancies. I can see the rationale for using antibiotics to help fight infections, as there is a certain sense that from an evolutionary perspective, these drugs and their structurally related cousins, synthesized in the laboratory, are perfectly designed for that function and purpose in microorganisms. But I am not convinced that they are or will be truly suitable, logical, or scientifically elegant

*** The Adriatic Sea got its name from the Roman Emperor Hadrian (76-138).**

cancer chemotherapy drugs. And a reminder that about 50 years ago when scientists talked about chemotherapy, they were talking most often about antibiotic therapy for infectious diseases!

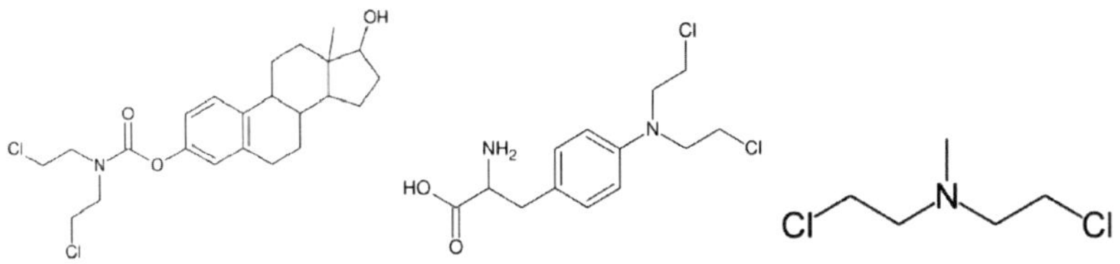

Estramustine, melphalan, and mechlorethamine: Nitrogen mustard gas derivatives. From gassing troops to treating patients with chemotherapy.

Unfortunately empiricism has once again prevailed above true understanding, which has led to an alphabet soup of regimens designed to "selectively" kill cancer cells.

AC, CMF, FEC, FAC, CEF, not to mention T-based regimens (Taxol or Taxotere), H-based regimens (Herceptin), X-based regimens (Xeloda), and so on.

The E by the way stands for epirubicin, another anthracycline like Adriamycin. And all I can say is it's only going to get crazier, unless we reconsider our approach. But I doubt it, and in fact the combinations of drugs will only become more confusing, and add the new "schedule du jour," dose density, which is the next "great" idea, based, I believe, on incorrect premises. So yes I am disappointed that we oncologists can be so stubborn and stupid.

Now back to Dr. Slamon's brave statement. For it suggests that right off, in patients with breast cancer, nearly 70-80%, treated with Adriamycin (and most likely epirubicin) for early-stage breast cancer, derive no benefit. Whether C (Cytoxan), or other chemotherapy alphabet letters help is not known, but my guess is that they do to a small extent (maybe 5-10% benefit). But in HER2-negative breast cancer, which I indicated represents the majority of cases, anthracycline-based regimens are no longer justified. And so our breast cancer thought leaders are busy creating new catchy acronyms for "novel" drug regimens. And even more amazingly, among HER2 positive breast cancers, only a small subset of patients benefit from anthracyclines. This population is around 5% of the total (those tumors that are HER2-positive and also overexpress an enzyme called topoisomerase IIA), so an incredible number of women with breast cancer have been treated with the absolutely wrong drug for more than 20 years.*

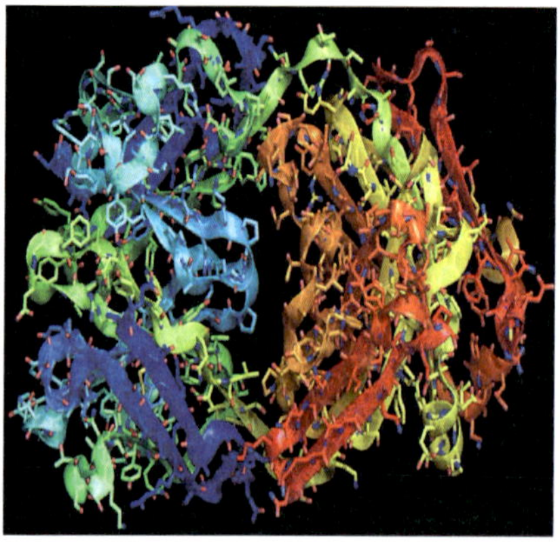

Herceptin structure. The treatment of cancer with very specific monoclonal antibodies that properly activate the immune system is one key element to rational therapy.

We'll talk about HER2 in detail later, but I'll tell you that it is a protein receptor that is a normal component of breast cells and many other cell types. In about 20-30% of breast cancers it is "overexpressed" in varying amounts. Inhibition of HER2 with the monoclonal antibody Herceptin (a billion dollar a year drug for Genentech), can help cure patients with early-stage breast cancer, in combination with other drugs, and it is also effective in prolonging the lives of women with metastatic disease, sometimes dramatically so. Even in carefully selected candidates with HER2-positive tumors, it's at best a coin-flip whether a meaningful or beneficial response will be seen. But at least Herceptin's creation was based on some thought, although when we speak of HER2-negative tumors, we are being disingenuous since the protein is present in relatively low numbers; 20,000 molecules per cell can be considered "negative."

* **We are getting a bit more scientific testing for topoisomerase II overexpression. Tests are now being performed in many hospitals. Breast cancer that overexpresses this enzyme should be "sensitive" to anthracycline chemotherapy, so at least there is some rationale for its continued use. The problem is we don't know whether other drug combinations are any better.**

And Herceptin can be dangerous to use (feel free to review its toxicity profile on the Genentech website). So, please be very skeptical when you hear about other new drugs with the catch-phrases like "revolutionary," "paradigm shift," "extraordinary" and similar hyperbole.

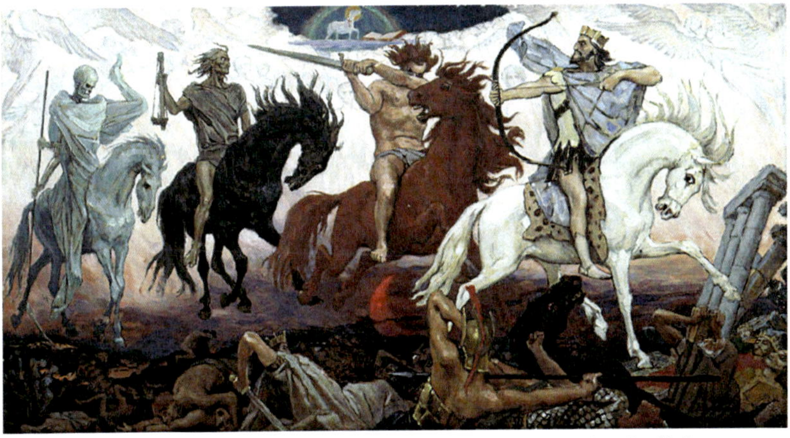

Apocalyptic vision of the way, to a large extent, (metaphorically) we treat cancer: Poisonous drugs, radiation, mutilating surgery, and the absence of faith in God all contribute to the mess we're in.

And with a "dose" of linguistic irony, as I end this essay, monoclonal antibodies (like Herceptin), can be conventionally abbreviated as Moab;* which leads us back to the beginning of biblical history. So we begin and end this essay with a cautionary tale, written by the Hand of God 4,000 years ago!!!

*** Over the last 30 years since the production of monoclonal antibodies the abbreviation changed from Moab to Mab but that would ruin the tenuous connections of this story!**

XVI. The Other Peyton

~~Science arose from poetry - when times change the two can meet again on a higher level as friends.~~ Johann Wolfgang von Goethe (1749-1832)

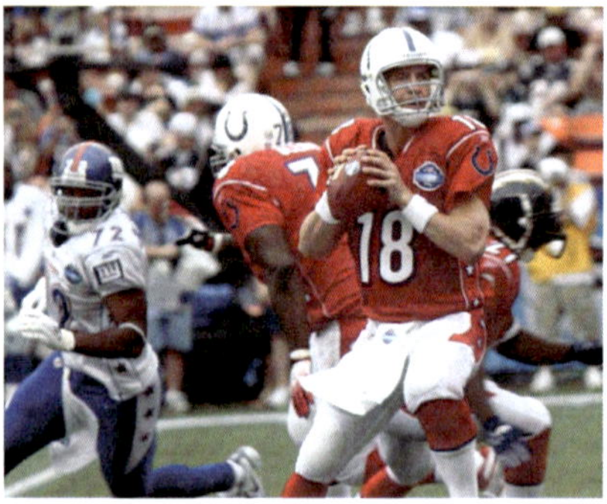

Peyton Manning: Super Bowl winner in 2007. His brother, Eli, won for the NY Giants in 2008.

With the NFL playoffs upon us as of this writing, everyone who follows this great game knows who Peyton is.

Peyton Manning is a future Hall of Fame quarterback for the Indianapolis Colts. For those readers who are less familiar with the game, he led his team to a Super Bowl victory in 2007 and just lost to the New Orleans Saints in 2010.*

To win a Super Bowl is a very difficult thing to do, and among millions of young athletes in this country it is considered a dream come true for athletic excellence.

But what about the nerds of the world?

And here lies the story of the other Peyton.

First, let us consider the nerd. The nerd is a term that somehow evolved into meaning someone who is extremely bright intellectually and has an intense focus on some pursuit such as computers, or science. He or she is typically a bookworm with few social skills. But did you know, among my nerd audience, that the word "nerd" was invented by Dr. Seuss? And that it had no meaning when first used by him in a children's book in 1950?

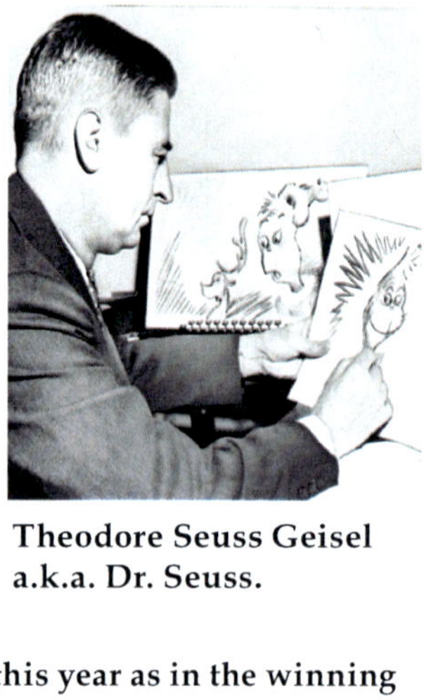

Theodore Seuss Geisel a.k.a. Dr. Seuss.

*** Homonymous irony: Peyton lost to Payton this year as in the winning coach Sean Payton.**

Or that Dr. Seuss (Theodor Seuss Geisel) was a Dartmouth College graduate? Or that he entered Oxford University for a PhD but never completed his doctorate*?

So what does this have to do with the other Peyton?

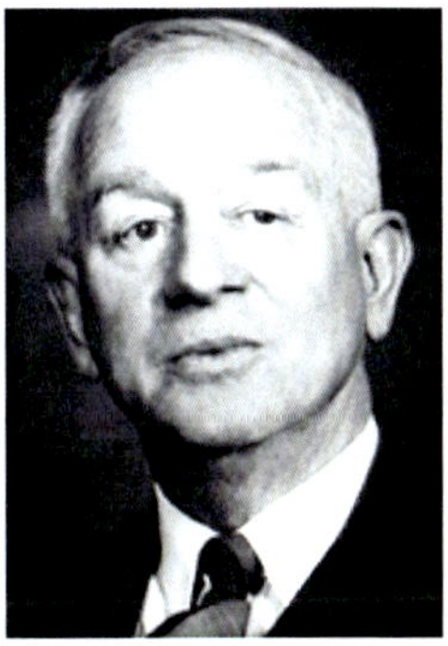

Peyton Rous, MD. We are lucky he didn't like being a Texas cowpoke more!

Well among nerds, the one prize above all others to aspire to is the Nobel Prize, which in 1966 was won by two men who shared equally in the cash payout (now around 1.5 million dollars). Charles Huggins won for understanding the importance of hormones in cancer and we'll talk more about him another time. And the other winner was Peyton Rous.

Peyton Rous was a meganerd. He was a native Texan who decided that being a cowboy was perhaps not the best use of his prodigious intellect, although he did participate (as a nerd would say) in a cattle drive as a young man.

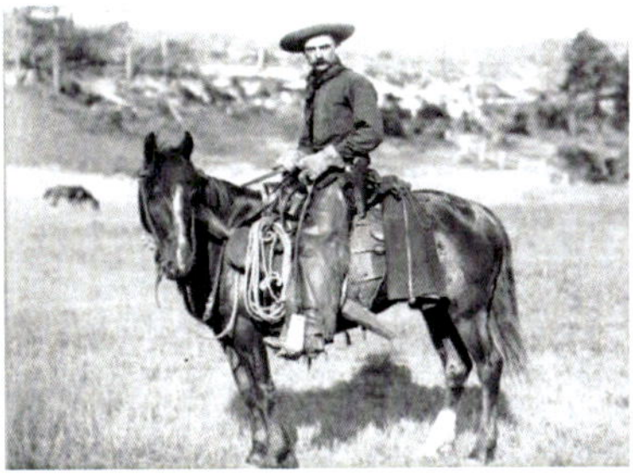

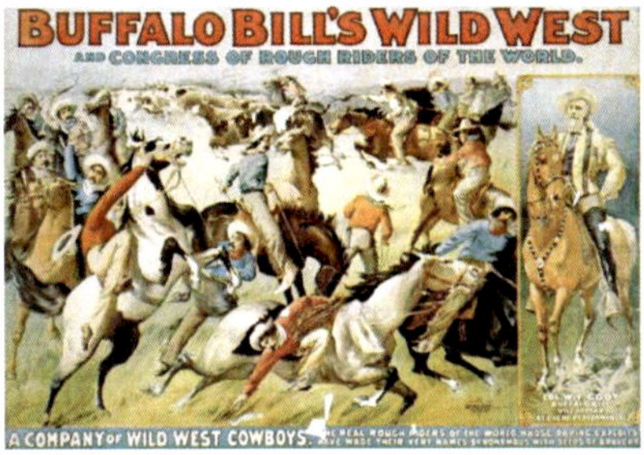

Dr. Rous chose to round up chickens and rabbits instead of cattle.

He eventually ended up at the Rockefeller Institute in New York, after graduating from Johns Hopkins Medical School. And he spent his entire scientific career there, mostly in the presence of chickens and rabbits.

What he discovered about 100 years ago is so important that it has changed the course of medicine in a way that could

*** His father was disappointed that he didn't get his doctorate, hence the nom de plume.**

be compared to the discovery of electricity. In other words, in a huge way!

He discovered that viruses can cause cancer!

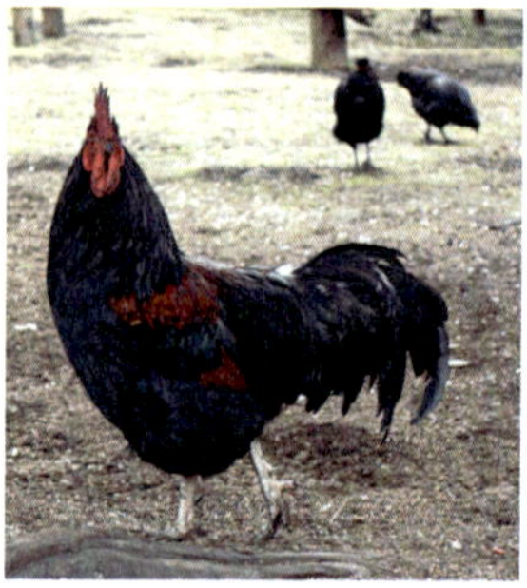

Lasso that chicken!

Working with chickens in 1911, he published a paper that described the transmission of a type of cancer called sarcoma which could be separated from the tumor cells and passed through the finest filters. (17)

He also studied rabbit tumors called papillomas which were also caused by viruses and in fact these papillomas are similar to papillomas that can occur in humans which are caused by the human papilloma virus (HPV) which can promote the development of cervical and other cancers. And now there are cancer vaccines, (Gardasil and Cervarix) approved for preventing HPV infection from ever occurring!

But I am getting ahead of myself in my "nerdsome" zeal.

As is so typical of great discoveries, in 1911 the "experts" laughed at Peyton Rous. And for 15 years or so they continued to laugh at his silly work with critters. But then they stopped laughing.

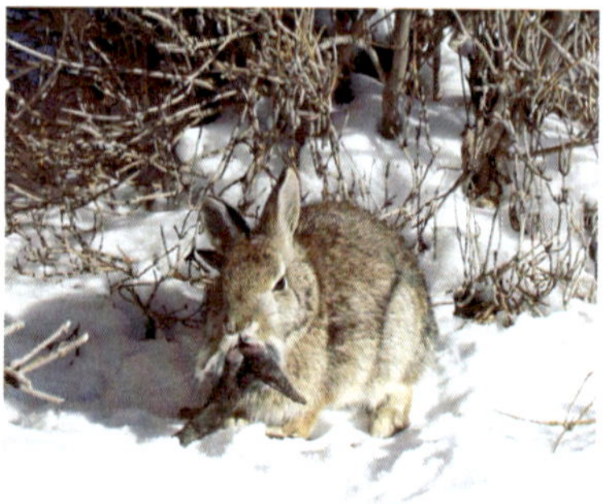

An incredible photo of a wild rabbit infected with a papilloma-virus similar to HPV. The weird growth by its mouth is a virally-induced tumor!

Finally in 1966 the ultimate nerd was honored by his peers with the Nobel Prize. This prize was created by another nerd, Alfred Nobel, who you might not want to laugh at since he invented TNT.

So when they talk about the Nobel Prize Ceremony being a "blast" they ain't kidding as they say in Texas.

And as my Texas friend Billy Bob says: "We'll be talkin' more about these cancer vaccines real soon."

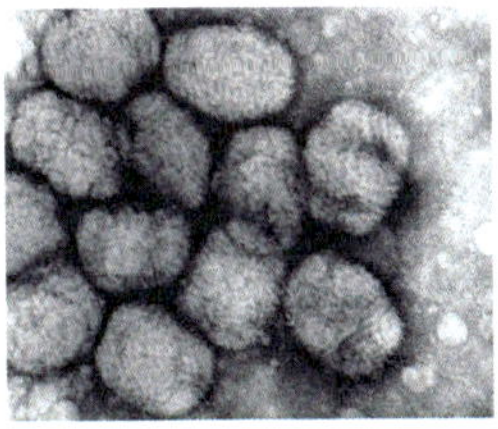

Smallpox.

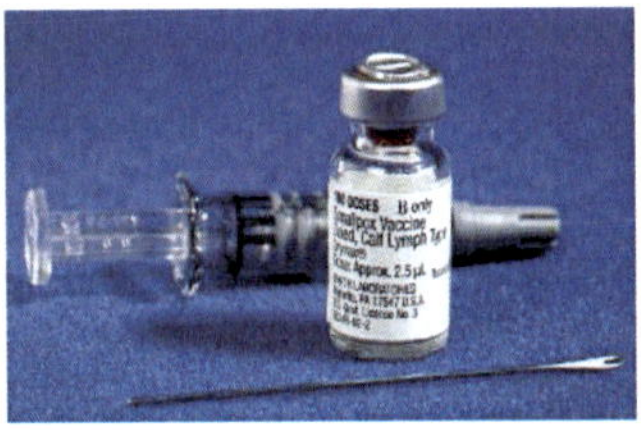

Smallpox vaccine.

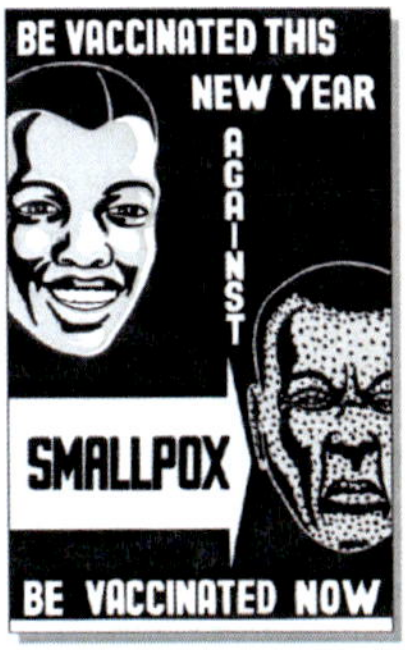
BE VACCINATED THIS
NEW YEAR
AGAINST
SMALLPOX
BE VACCINATED NOW

Small pox vaccination poster.

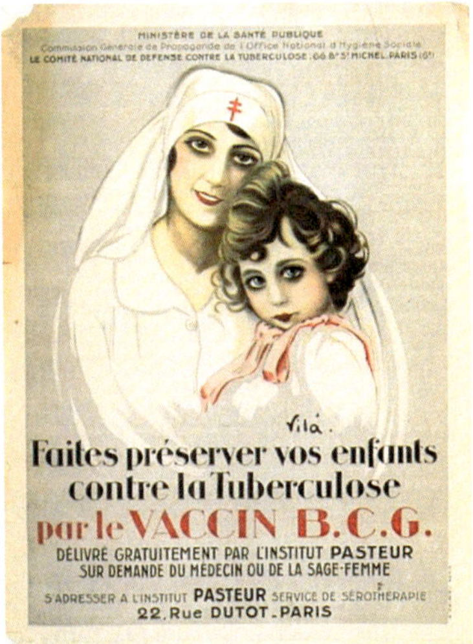
MINISTÈRE DE LA SANTÉ PUBLIQUE
LE COMITÉ NATIONAL DE DÉFENSE CONTRE LA TUBERCULOSE
Vila.
Faites préserver vos enfants
contre la Tuberculose
par le VACCIN B.C.G.
DÉLIVRÉ GRATUITEMENT PAR L'INSTITUT PASTEUR
SUR DEMANDE DU MÉDECIN OU DE LA SAGE-FEMME
S'ADRESSER A L'INSTITUT PASTEUR SERVICE DE SÉROTHÉRAPIE
22, Rue DUTOT . PARIS

Vaccination against infectious diseases has benefited mankind in incalculable ways, and will continue to do so in the 21st century. Bill Gates, through his wonderful foundation, has just earmarked $10 billion dollars for this endeavor.

XVII. Microtruth

~~Of all lies, art is the least untrue.~~ Gustave Flaubert (1821-1880)

I am sitting in a lecture hall about 35 years ago and our organic chemistry professor at Queens College in New York, Dr. Axelrod, is handing out exams, and I'm praying that I can survive this ordeal. Dr. Axelrod was short and squat and terrifying. His gaze was penetrating, with his glass eye participating in a totally intimidating visage.

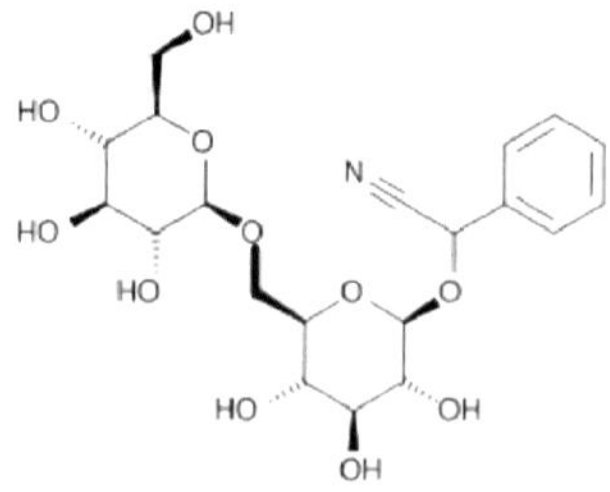

Laetrile is not the answer.

The last question was about laetrile or amygdalin. It's also incorrectly called vitamin B17 and it's sometimes derived from apricot pits, in a chemical extraction process that leads to the isolation of a sugar molecule distantly related to glucose, like one is distantly related to a never-seen crazy uncle, who is whispered about at holiday gatherings. For laetrile is a glycoside that carries a cyanide moiety which when released kills cells and sometimes people from cyanide poisoning.

The question involved the synthesis of amygdalin from a sugar precursor, using various catalytic processes. By a stroke of luck I got the question right, but there was no future for me in chemistry.

In the 1970's the laetrile controversy peaked, and various citizens formed political action organizations to allow the use of this drug in treating cancer. Lawsuits were filed in federal courts and the highest levels of government were involved in deciding the fate of laetrile in this country. For those readers interested in this fascinating story, go to the Quackwatch website, and access a superb article by Benjamin Wilson, MD: "The Rise and Fall of Laetrile."

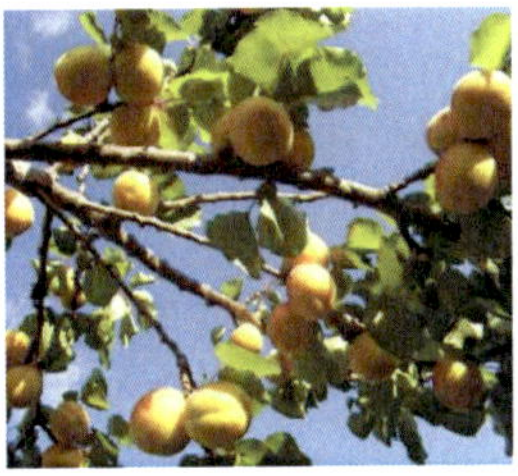

Apricot tree.

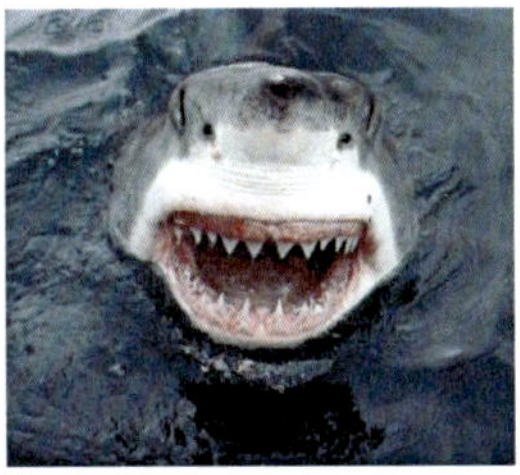

Shark.
"People believe what they want to believe."

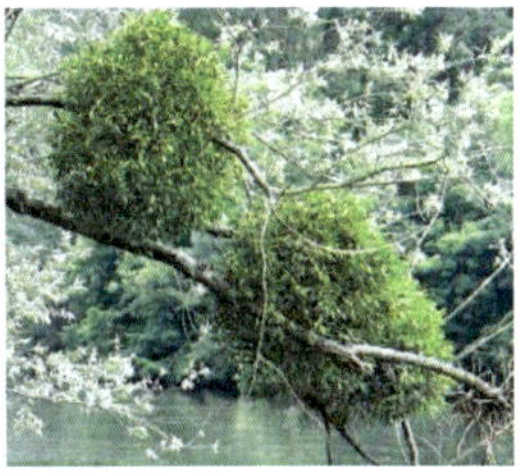

Mistletoe.

For laetrile is the poster child for ineffective chemotherapy drugs that continue to be used in treating desperate patients with advanced cancer, despite having been shown to have no objective benefit. Other examples we will talk briefly about are shark cartilage (Neovastat), and mistletoe extract (Iscador).*

On a more personal note, a patient with metastatic colon cancer came to see me several years ago. She and her husband had decided to travel to Mexico for laetrile therapy, where it is approved, although it turns out that in Montana and Indiana, laetrile therapy is still legal... They "do it better in Mexico," according to her. And she wants my opinion.

Should I say?: 1) That's a great idea.
2) That's a stupid idea.
3) That's both a great and a stupid idea.

I will not reveal my response to maintain an air of mystery. She and her husband had already decided what the best course of action was for them, based on their belief systems. All we can do is wish them well and offer to help in any way we can.

So they went to Mexico, she was treated at a cancer clinic there, having a catheter placed in her hepatic vein, and received a combination of laetrile, 5-Fluorouracil, high-dose vitamin B12, and other "vitamins." Five months later, she returned to see me,

*** A recent journey led me past Mistletoe State Park, near Augusta, Georgia. I doubt hiking there as opposed to a different State Park has any added chemopreventive benefits.**

and she said that she felt much better, although she had lost 40 more pounds and looked more like a skeleton than a person.

Three months later, the obituary described "her brave fight against cancer."

How are we to interpret these events? First, she received a chemotherapy regimen that included 5-Fluorouracil, which for more than 50 years has been used in treating solid tumors, and remains one of the mainstays in colon cancer. Second, hepatic vein (or artery) infusions have been used with modest success in this country in people with liver metastases. So the issue really is whether adding laetrile and other things was beneficial in prolonging her life and making her feel better. Despite the results of clinical trials designed to answer this question demonstrating no statistical benefit in adding laetrile to conventional chemotherapy (18), we will never know whether it helped (or hurt) this unfortunate woman. Because the added dimension to our calculus is the idea, which is a powerful force in human nature that she believed laetrile helped make her feel better and extended her life by precious months. This may have also been a great blessing to her family. Then the dilemma is: "If one believes that a drug helps them, we can never entirely refute their claim."

In a conversation not too long ago with my mentor Dr. Lloyd Old at Sloan-Kettering Institute, he shared with me his observations about the laetrile controversy which created such a tremendous amount of anger between patient groups supporting its use, and scientists and physicians against it. He suggested to his colleagues at the time that the best approach was to have both sides meet for a free exchange of thoughts, but of course this never happened, despite it being the most logical approach.

This reminded me of an earlier conversation with Dr. Old (who, as you know from previous essays, I consider the world's leading cancer biologist and founder of modern cancer immunology) in which he quoted the brilliant logician and philosopher Alfred North Whitehead: "It is more important for an idea to be interesting, than it is to be true."

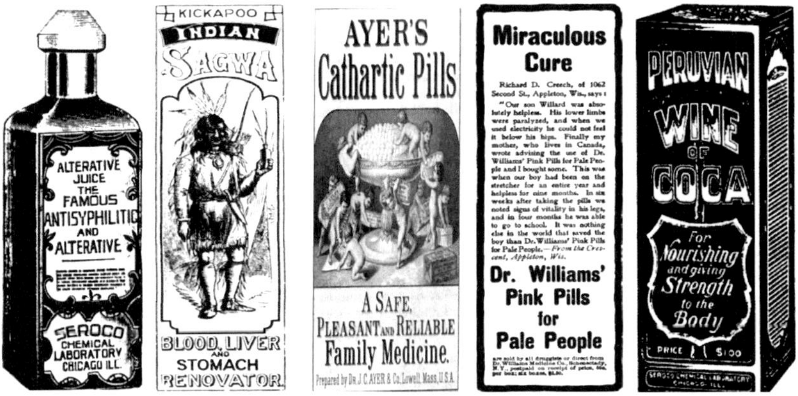

Patent medicines and their absurd claims.

So now, the title of this essay will be defined, "Microtruth": An extremely miniscule truth encased and shrouded in falsehood.

Laetrile kills cancer cells, and sometimes it seems to help people who use it in attacking their cancer. The microtruth of laetrile is that it is no better than the most amazing, and controversial, alternative therapy ever invented: the "placebo." For the placebo is the mysterious drug that shouldn't help anyone feel better or control the symptoms of any disease, and yet in countless studies, by reputable investigators, it does just that. Sometimes it works better than the drug supposed to be more effective, sometimes less so, but we always assume as scientists and physicians that a placebo is a useless treatment. But this is also a microtruth, because we ignore the fact that for admittedly mysterious reasons, it does help some people with cancer and other diseases, and whether this placebo-effect is a consequence of neuroimmunology, spontaneous regression (which might have occurred anyway), or an act of Almighty God, it doesn't matter as long as people get better.

The problem with laetrile, shark cartilage and mistletoe, is that as Julius Caesar said: "People believe what they want to believe."

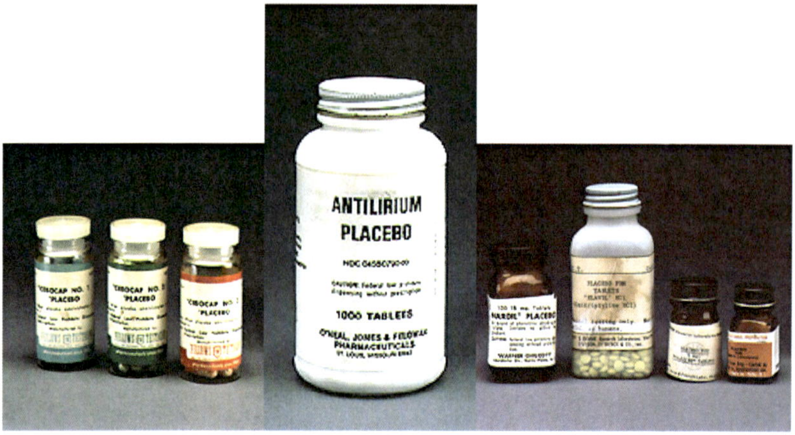

The placebo is still a powerful and perhaps now underutilized "medicine."

So when reports of the ability of these drugs to influence immune function or inhibit angiogenesis are published (19, 20), desperate patients will do desperate things. For the issue is really not what works by whatever mechanism we believe is relevant, but what works best, with the least toxicity. At the risk of a heretical thought, one approach (although it is considered by many to be unethical) would be to give patients a placebo, claiming it is a substance that might help them. Rather than summarily dismissing this silly idea, consider what physicians were doing for thousands of years, before effective therapies for any disease existed!

For the microtruth in the use of conventional chemotherapy in oncology is that it has consistently achieved a meaningful benefit in patients with advanced cancer. And if that statement were true, the use of unconventional, ineffective and toxic drugs like Vitamin B17, Neovastat, and Iscador would never occur.

XVIII. When is Breast Cancer, Which is Not Breast Cancer, Breast Cancer?

~~"An expert is a man who has made all the mistakes which can be made in a very narrow field."~~ Niels Bohr (1885-1962)

I will repeat the headline of this essay as a point of emphasis, lest you think it is a typographical error or I have gone mad.

When is breast cancer, which is not breast cancer, breast cancer?

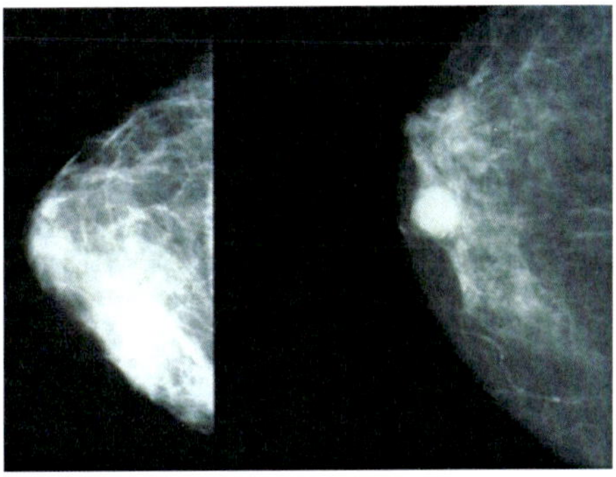

An experienced radiologist can correctly interpret routine mammograms about 75% of the time. Notice the dense but normal breast on the left.

Let us begin with a woman who undergoes her yearly mammogram. It shows a suspicious abnormality in the right breast, less than a centimeter in size, with microcalcifications, that the radiologist, ever diligent, recommends: "a biopsy of this abnormality, possibly under ultrasound guidance, as it cannot be detected by clinical palpation."

The woman, who is now a "patient," is frantic, as are her husband and immediate family. She is 50 years old and just ran a marathon last week. She does everything right and is constantly trying to decrease her risk of cancer, by eating well, exercising, and anything else believed to help.

A biopsy is performed on a Friday afternoon. Everything goes well from a technical standpoint. As she leaves to go home she asks the radiologist when the diagnosis will be back. He indicates that it won't be formally interpreted by the pathologist until MONDAY! Now she is really upset about waiting and, being a type AAA personality, she calls her primary care doctor to complain (and see if things can be speeded up, which they can't in a small community hospital with limited histology technicians to prepare slides.)

She waits in a vigil-like setting for about 4,000 minutes (72 hours), and is called by her primary physician with good news. He tells her that the breast mass that was biopsied is called lobular carcinoma in situ and her chance of being cured with just an excisional biopsy performed by a surgeon is about 100%.

Now she calls her brother-in-law who is a PhD scientist at a famous university. He calls one of the world's experts in LCIS (lobular carcinoma in situ) who tells him that the term lobular carcinoma in situ is no longer used by the world's leading experts. Instead we call it lobular neoplasia, and yes it's a tumor (neoplasia) but not cancer (carcinoma). But some experts still call it carcinoma in situ, but he's not friends with them because of this dispute.

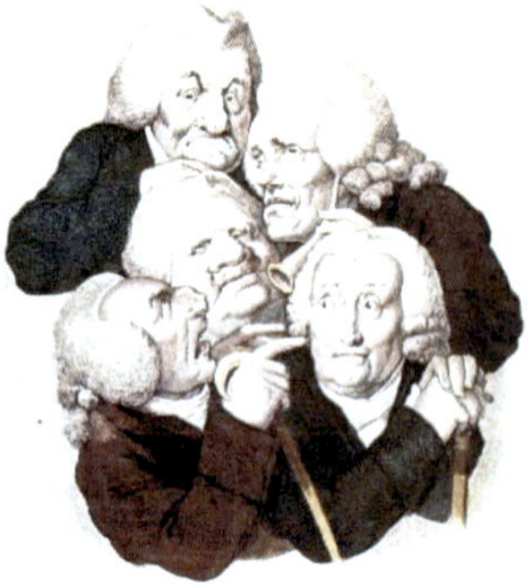

Cancer experts like to disagree with each other.

So her brother-in-law calls other experts and reviews the world literature and discovers several areas of scientific controversy.

1) Lobular neoplasia (formerly lobular carcinoma in situ) does not always need to be surgically excised. (21)

2) Lobular carcinoma in situ (now lobular neoplasia) does need to be surgically excised. (22)

3) Lobular neoplasia (formerly lobular carcinoma in situ) is a benign lesion that is associated with an increased risk of developing breast cancer in either breast, but by itself probably has no malignant potential. (23)

4) Lobular carcinoma in situ can develop into invasive lobular carcinoma. (24, 25)

So if you are not somewhat confused by all this, you probably need to read it again, since it is Very Confusing.

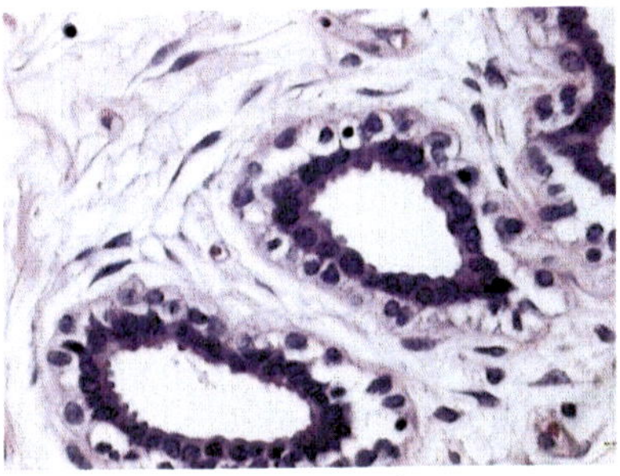

Normal breast tissue.

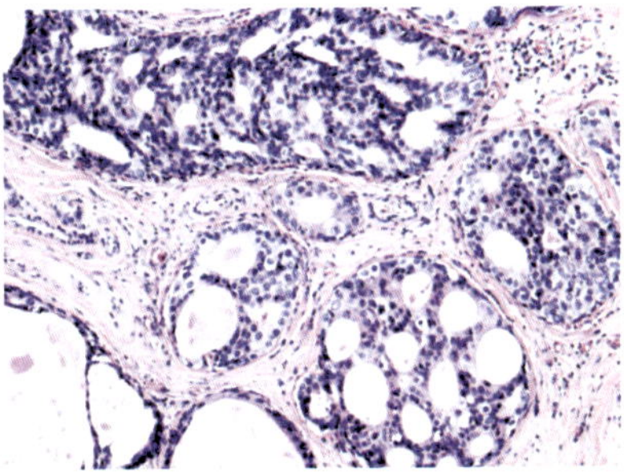

DCIS (ductal carcinoma in situ).

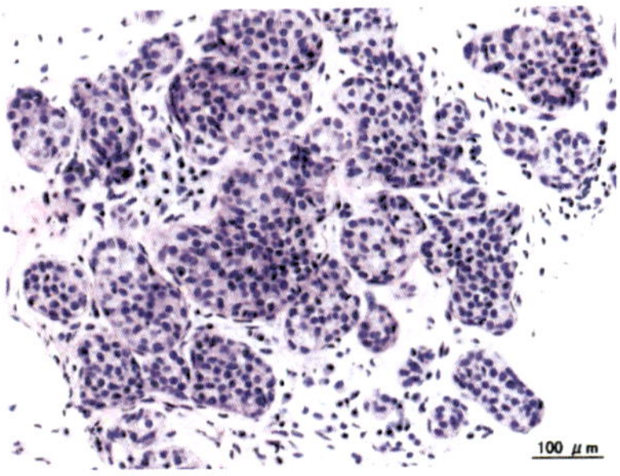

Invasive lobular carcinoma of breast.

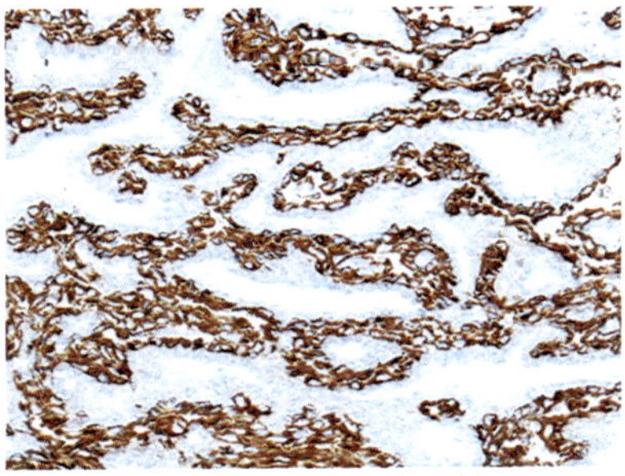

Intraductal papilloma of breast.

Even the most experienced pathologists can disagree about when breast cancer is breast cancer.

And hence, the perfectly appropriate and, if I may say, clever title of this essay.

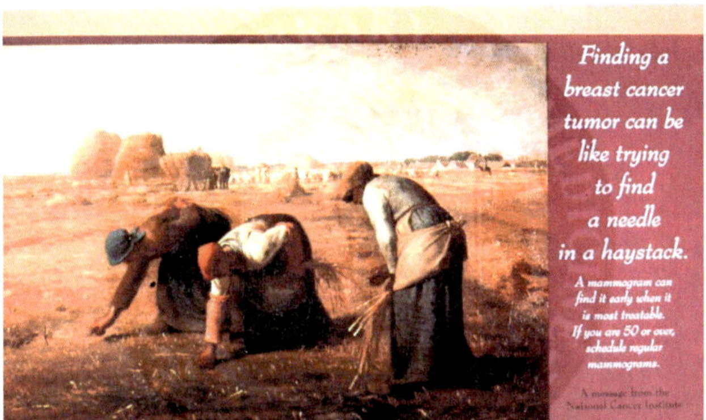
Finding a
breast cancer
tumor can be
like trying
to find
a needle
in a haystack.
A mammogram can
find it early when it
is most treatable.
If you are 50 or over,
schedule regular
mammograms.

Even large lobular carcinomas can be missed on mammography because of their insidious pattern of spread.

And don't worry, we'll be talking a lot about all sorts of confusing things in medicine in the future!

XIX. Quantum Oncology

~~"The key to wisdom is this - constant and frequent questioning... for by doubting we are led to question and by questioning we arrive at the truth."
Peter Abelard (1079-1142)

Let's start with an assumption: We know not what we do.

We turn on the lights and through a series of physico-chemical processes light is created, we are able to perceive this, and it is good.

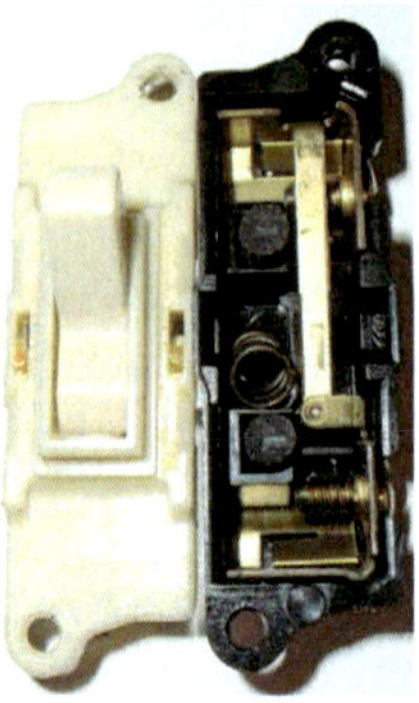

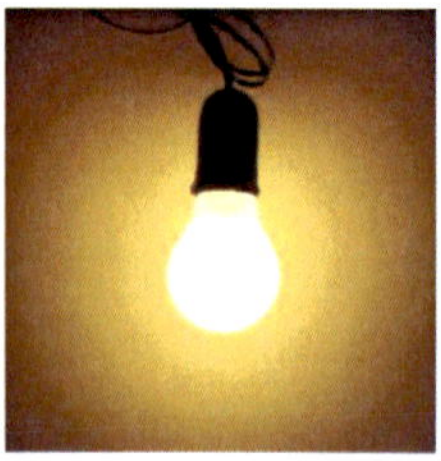

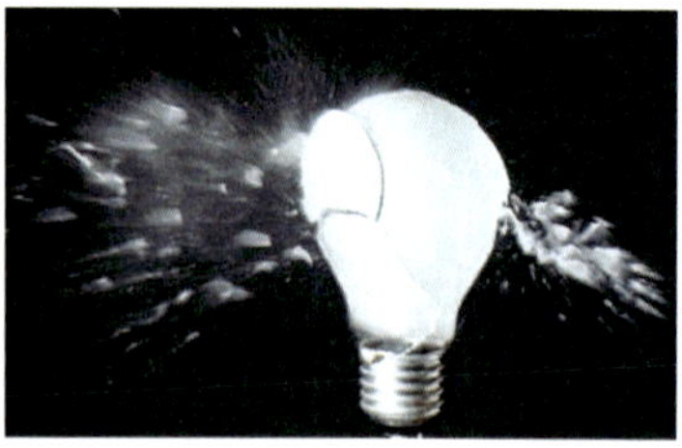

This explains everything. There will be a quiz later.

The universal constant in this activity is do something, and something else happens. Now I'm not pretending to be Newton, Maxwell, Faraday, Edison, Bohr, or Einstein. I'm just pretending to be an oncologist who spends time thinking about why things are the way they are, or seem to be. I'm a dreamer, so I like to dream. But the Monster.com job website has no positions in that capacity, yet, so I'm forced to consider other methods of satisfying my curiosity, like being a physician and writing this stuff.

But, maybe Poe was right when he said: "What we see or seem is but a dream within a dream."

Now I don't want to speculate about the meaning of life when I turn on a light, I just want it to work. If it doesn't, I'm irritated, having absolutely no mechanical ability to repair anything. Switch the switch and no light. Now what? First, jiggle it a few times. Next, check the light bulb by untwisting it, and shaking it; if it is blackened, and the filament makes a kind of ping sound, we are on to something! Next, (assuming other light sources are available), find a stinkin' light bulb. And so on. If there is no light in the house then the algorithm changes, for now we must consider the dreaded fuse box, electrical wiring, power outages, and other cataclysmic events.

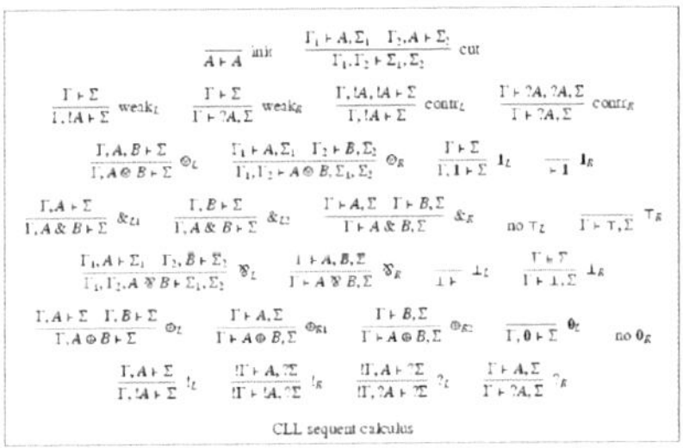

This will help us when the light won't go on!

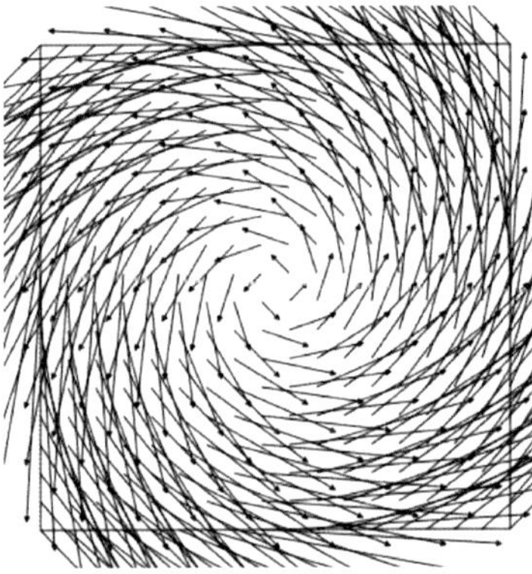

I don't need to know about electrons, impedance, Ohm's law, the Pauli exclusion principle, Heisenberg's uncertainty theory, the Schroedinger wave equation, or how anything works. Spin, vibration, angular momentum, velocity, and charge have no meaning to me now. When I studied these esoteric subjects in college I thought that I could make them a part of my intellectual life and help me understand how to apply them in some fashion or form in my work in medicine. But, forget about it!

What I do remember about college is: Pinball machines (Dimension was my favorite, even with one weak flipper), which allowed me to pass time rather than attend boring classes; foosball, where I could be humiliated by players much better than me. Other achievements: Working in the rathskeller as a short-order cook where I could flirt with girls; loading lead blocks and moving them to some other place at the atomic accelerator; washing glassware in a biochemistry lab; trolling for algae in a lake...

I failed structural chemistry (I could not derive the Schroedinger wave equation), but loved the squiggly integral lines.

Being told by my chemistry professor after he wrote on my exam: "Please see me." (Other classmates had things written like: "Great job." "Keep up your high standards.") "Cliff, (pause for effect), have you considered other majors besides chemistry?"

I just wanted to go to medical school.

So I now propose an idea which, if better developed and testable, would be considered a theory. And it ain't gonna be me who does that!

Equation 1: Time + toxic chemicals (carcinogens) + viruses + genetic instability = cancer.

Equation 2: Time + cancer = more cancer.

Equation 3: Time + cancer + cancer immunity = less cancer.

Equation 4: Probability of cancer as a life-threatening disease = Equation 1 + 2 + 3.

Equation 5: Equations 1 + 2 + 3 + 4 are all determined by the laws of Quantum Oncology.

Definition: Quantum Oncology - The study of cancer development based on the principles of quantum mechanics.

We are all basically atoms, which should obey the laws of physics. But the problem is the mathematical equations of quantum physics are inadequate to describe complicated atomic structures like genes and proteins. Not being smart enough to understand them in the first place may now work to my advantage! For it frees me from worrying about the details, like, "Why don't the equations balance," and other nerdy comments.

When people get cancer, let's use lung cancer as an example, why is it that there may be a primary tumor in the right lung in one patient, which has spread to a few local (hilar) lymph nodes, and a rib, right pelvis, and one spot in the left lobe of the liver? And in another patient with a right lung tumor (similar histology and primary size and location), which is in regional (mediastinal) lymph nodes, three spots in the liver (two on right, one on left), and a solitary spot in the right temporal lobe of the brain? And I could present a thousand examples or clinical vignettes of this sort.

So why does cancer start in one place and not the other? Why does it spread in cases of advanced or metastatic disease, to different places and not other places? It is probably not just a case of "soil and seed," which is a theory that's been around for more than 100 years. Nor, can things be easily explained by the failure of local or regional immunity (which I used to believe).

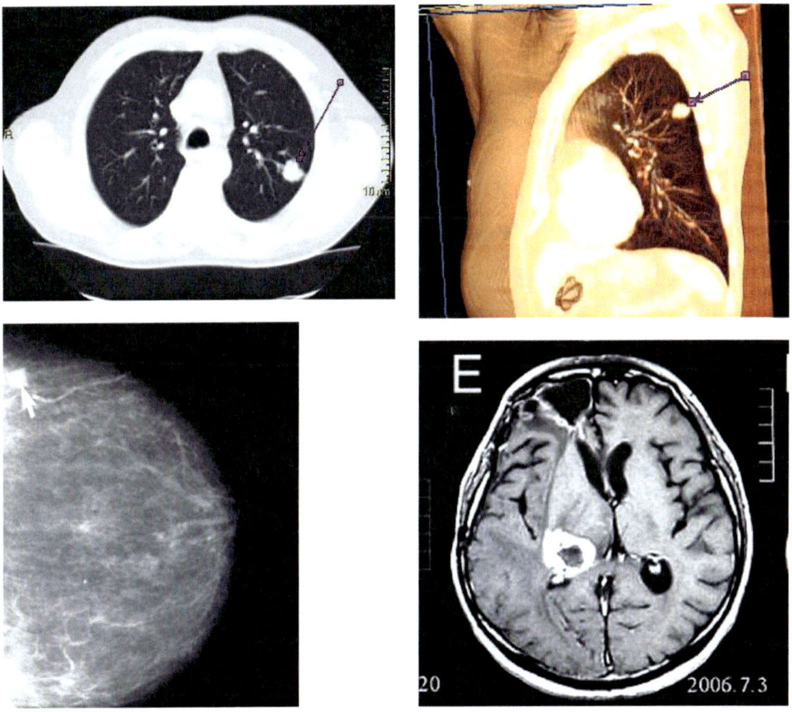

For the most part, there are no adequate explanations for why cancer occurs in one location and not another, beyond probabilistic considerations.

The reasons for cancer development as outlined in the equations are simply that random events occur that cannot be predicted with absolute certainty due to the same physical principles that make it impossible to accurately predict the location of an electron or any other atomic or subatomic particle from which we are ultimately composed of, in the form of proteins, lipids, nucleic acids, organelles, cells, structures, organs, creatures....

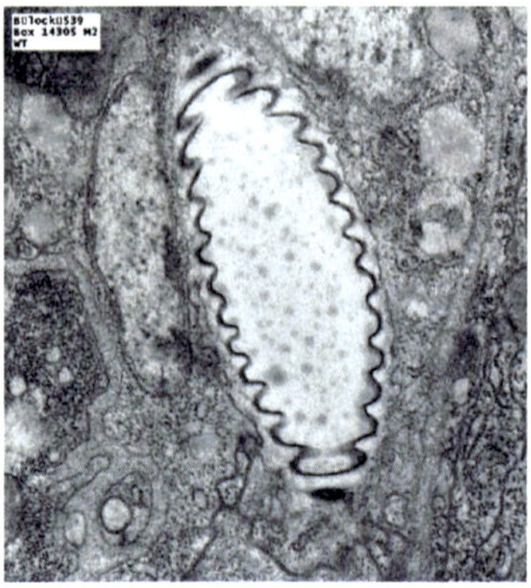

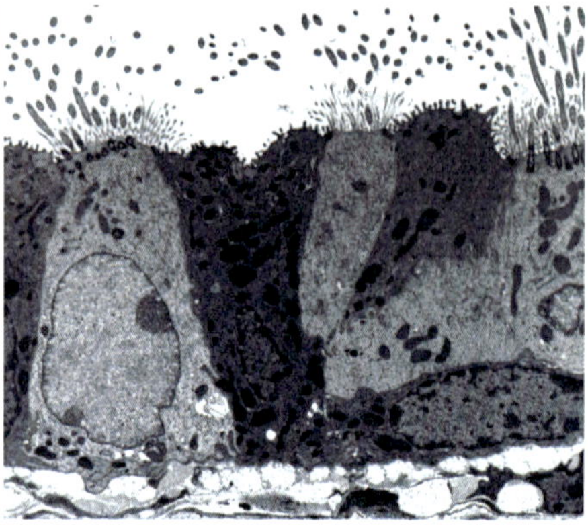

Taenidiae **Lung epithelium**

Transcendental cellular complexity.

So why should we expect to know precisely where cancer will start, and go to, when we can't figure out where an electron is (the best we can do is describe its cloud-like distribution), which along with a gazillion other electrons, allowed me to turn on the light in my house and write this essay.

For the wheel of cancer fortune turns, and where it ends up, nobody knows!

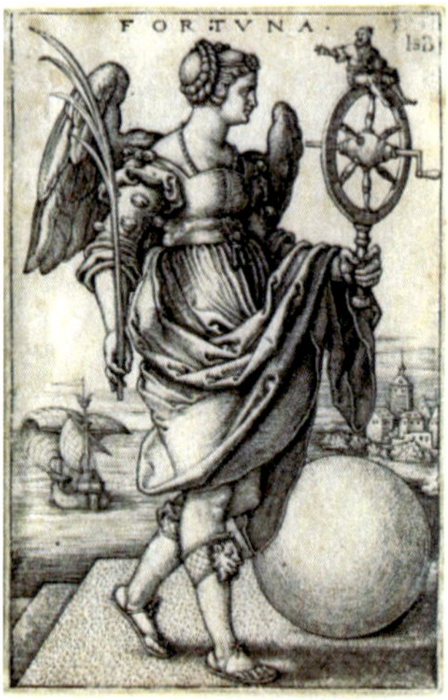

Fortune and her wheel.

XX. The Nude Molecular Biologist

~~Do what you will, this world's a fiction and is made up of contradiction."~~
William Blake (1757-1827)

Can the absurdity of the human condition, of which we are prisoners of sorts, be explained by a story about a west coast hippie who changed the course of social history?

I doubt it, but let's try anyway.

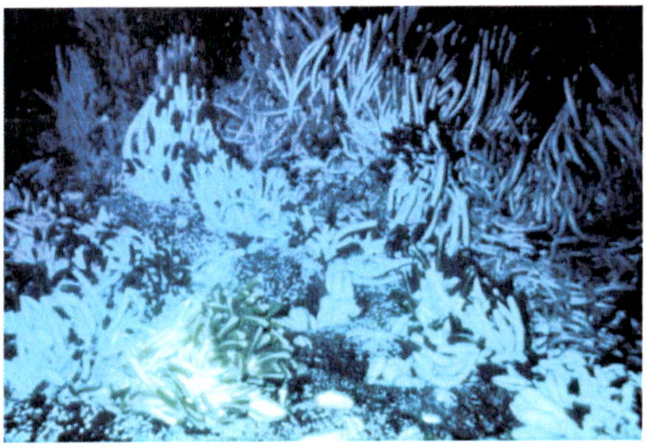

A hydrothermal vent where tubeworms live off of thermophilic bacteria in the "cracks of hell."

From out of the depths of creation, within the cracks of Hell are spewed methane gas and brimstone in the form of various sulfur compounds that are released in hydrothermal vents called black smokers. These geological events occur thousands of feet below the earth's ocean surface, in the form of underground eruptions of magma at incredible temperature and pressure. And there we of course find some life form that has evolved to survive and thrive, which is eaten by other things and so on.

But how can a man, unjustly accused of a crime such as murder and incarcerated for 25 years, find hope in these observations?

And how can a cancer patient breathe a sigh of relief from a test that was indirectly created by some fantastic bacteria that can live at the edge of the abyss?

And how can an LSD-tripping molecular biologist be part of this puzzle?

And what does this have to do with Ulysses S. Grant, our 18th president, and Theodore Roosevelt, our 26th president?

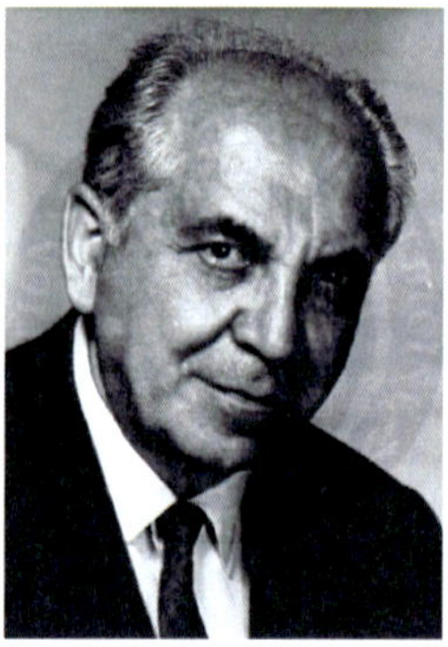

Ludwik Gross, MD, discoverer of endogenous retroviruses.

Or a Jewish physician/scientist/ Polish emigre/VA employee who discovered endogenous retroviruses, which led to discovery of the HIV virus?

Let's begin at the beginning of time when ancient bacteria called extremophiles figured out a way of living under "extreme" conditions. Under tons of pressure and heat, they are happy and are capable of using methane and sulfur compounds to provide their energy requirements in a process called chemosynthesis, and other things eat them, such as the Pompeii worm (great name).

In studying these bacteria, which are also called thermophiles (heat lovers), in hydrothermal vents and in other places with similar geologic activity such as the hot springs of Yellowstone National Park, scientists about 35 years ago found that various enzymes that the bacteria produced functioned best at temperatures that could fry an

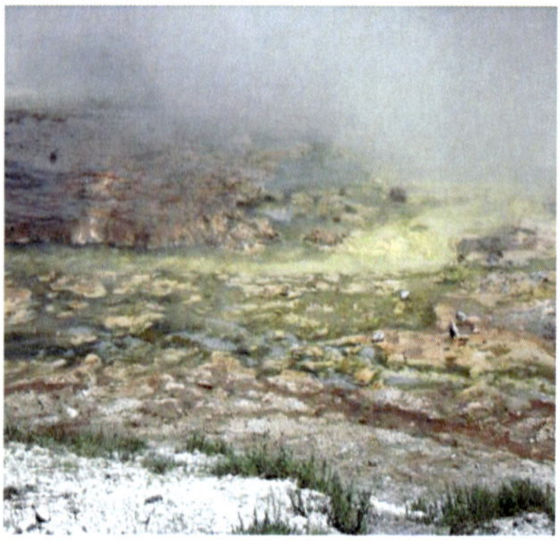

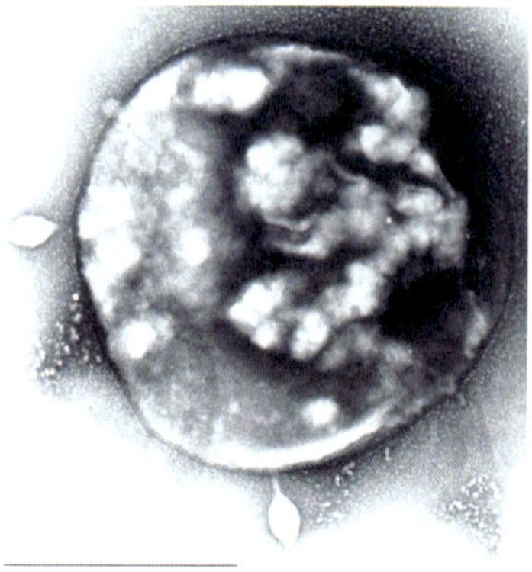

Yellowstone geyser where thermophilic bacteria like sulfolobus live. The protrusions on sulfolobus are specific viruses which can infect it!

egg. Yellowstone National Park was first dedicated in 1872 by President Grant and then President T. Roosevelt had the vision to create the National Parks Service around 1900, to further protect this treasured land where scientific discoveries could be made in a pristine setting.

So the nude molecular biologist could have his (perhaps) LSD-influenced vision.

For Kary Mullis in 1983, (in 1998 the author of the autobiography: "Dancing Naked in the Mind Field") inadvertently figured out a way to save the unjustly accused and imprisoned, among other things.

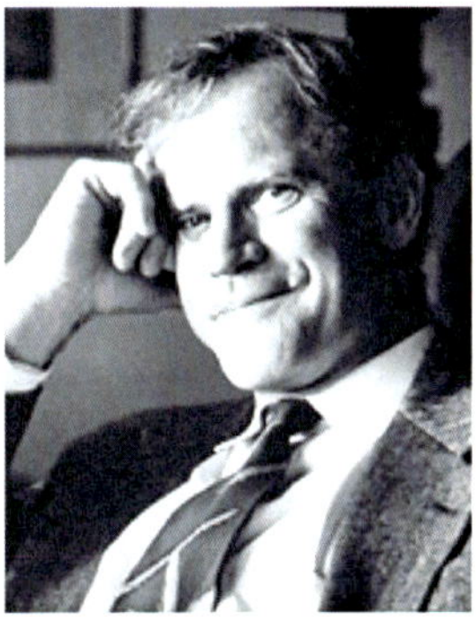

Kary Mullis, Ph.D. His discovery of PCR has changed the way criminal evidence is analyzed and sometimes freed the innocent.

He realized that he could exploit other scientist's discoveries of heat-loving enzymes such as the DNA polymerase isolated from Thermus aquaticus, in creating a method called PCR or the polymerase chain reaction. There are now about 20 variations of this reaction which use high heat in some of the steps to create amplified copies of DNA or sometimes RNA.

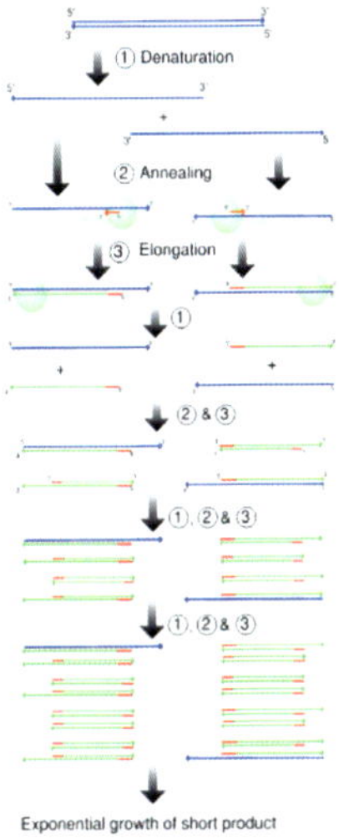

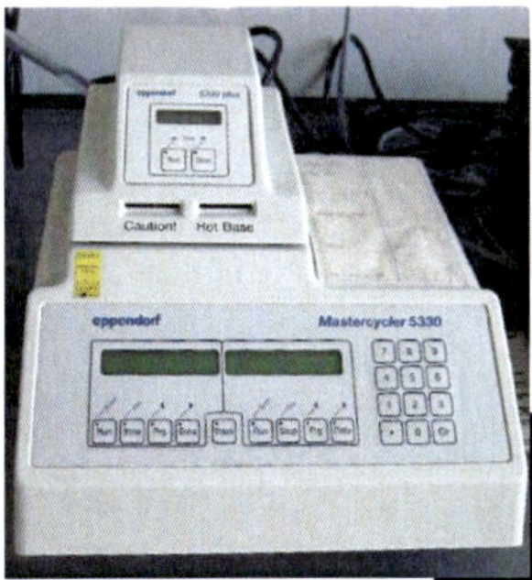

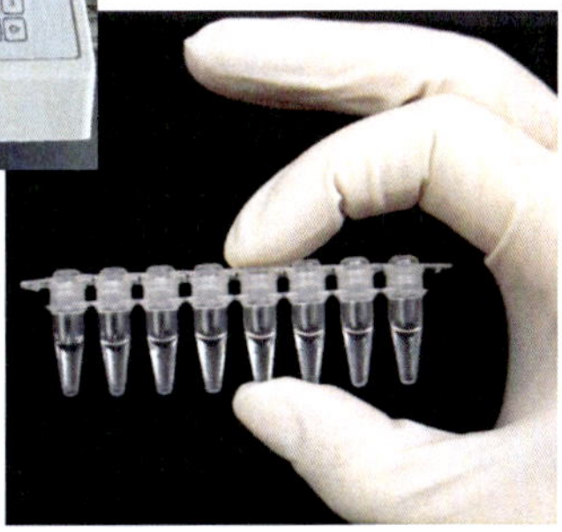

PCR (polymerase chain reaction) will continue to have a profound impact on future scientific discoveries in cancer research.

Not only did Dr. Mullis win the Nobel Prize in Chemistry in 1993, but his method (PCR) and the Thermus aquaticus polymerase were honored by the journal Science Magazine in 1989, in its augural award: "Molecule of the Year!"

Without realizing all the implications of his brilliant invention, Dr. Mullis has helped to free hundreds of prisoners who were unjustly accused of terrible crimes such as rape and murder. By testing minute amounts of blood or semen, scientists can use PCR as a forensic tool, to see if the DNA matches the accused or not.*

Another PCR test is called RT-PCR. The RT stands for reverse transcriptase which is an enzyme found in RNA viruses that infect people and animals and cause all sorts of diseases including cancer, leukemia, and AIDS. The discovery of this enzyme changed what was called the paradigm of molecular biology and led to Nobel Prizes for Howard Temin, David Baltimore, and Renato Dulbeco in 1975.

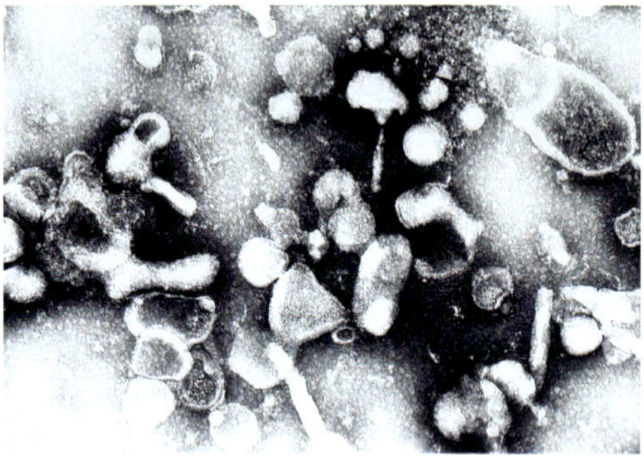

Feline lukemia virus is a retrovirus. Now, a vaccine can prevent infection from being transmitted between cats.

These viruses are called retroviruses and the man who really understood that viruses could cause cancer through natural infection and transmission from parent to offspring was a man named Ludwik Gross. As we alluded to before, he escaped Poland before the Nazis could kill him for being Jewish and served in the US Army medical corps, and he eventually ended up at a Bronx, NY VA hospital where he worked alone for years in a one-room lab, studying a mouse leukemia virus, eventually named after him.

And like Peyton Rous, and the terrible reception that he had from his colleagues, few believed Dr. Gross when he said in 1954 that viruses could cause cancer in mammals or humans. (26)

The Gross leukemia virus is an RNA virus (retrovirus) that can integrate into the cellular genome by activating an

*** This test can also help convict criminals who might otherwise escape the judicial system.**

enzyme it carries with it (described before) called reverse transcriptase and, just like HIV, cause a terrible consequences. Now there are several drugs like zidovudine, which can control HIV infection by inhibiting this reverse transcriptase enzyme, often prolonging patients' lives for many years.

Dr. Gross and other scientists made an equally profound discovery: Retroviruses, millions of years ago, were already part of the DNA of many if not all creatures.

In other words we humans are already part virus!

To that issue we will return later.

What about the cancer patient with melanoma, for instance, who has been told that the cancer was completely removed and the lymph nodes negative? Does that mean a cure? Are there other tests to tell whether the cancer will return?

For those questions RT-PCR may help us to see who will likely be cured with surgery. For it can detect a tiny fragment of melanoma DNA in the blood (in the form of messenger RNA) which is ultimately amplified and copied millions of times by RT-PCR.

By isolating a speck of RNA from 1 cell out of 10 million cells, RT-PCR, using the most specific and sensitive probes, may someday reassure patients with early-stage melanoma that they have been truly cured of this potentially horrible disease. Unfortunately we are not there yet, as various research groups have reported conflicting results to date, but I believe my prediction will come true in coming years (27-30).

So to summarize this crazy trip, from the depths of Hell to justice and peace of mind, a quote from William Blake, who was read by the famous philosopher Aldous Huxley, who wrote of "The Doors of Perception" after ingesting LSD, and encouraged other "minds."

Attraction and Repulsion.
Reason and Energy.
Love and Hate.
Are Necessary to Human Existence.

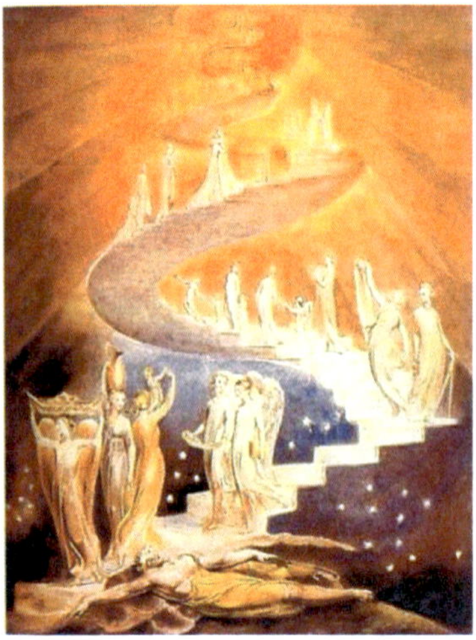

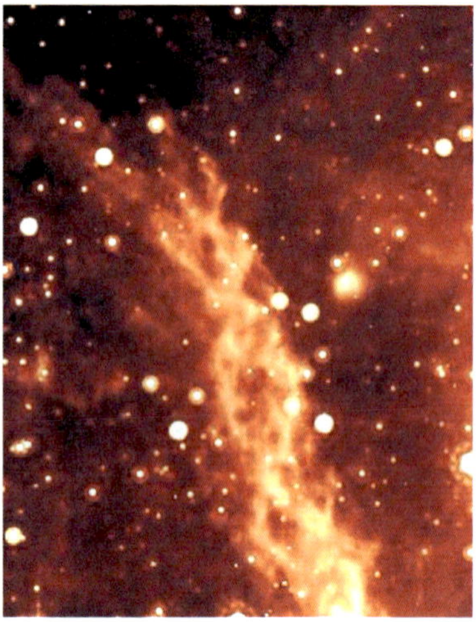

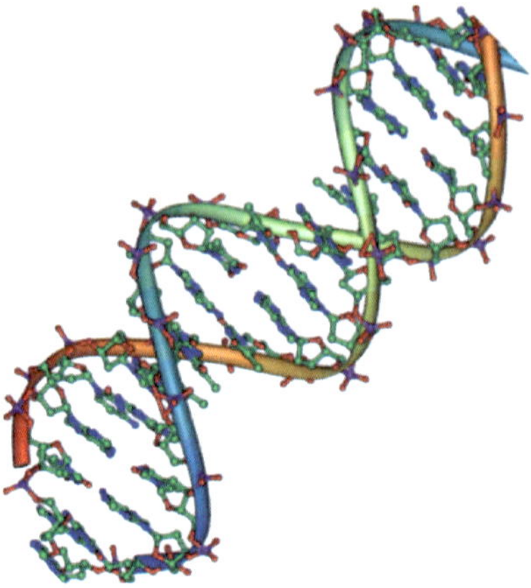

William Blake's conception of Jacob's ladder and DNA nebula, with or without hallucinogens, bear some resemblance to the DNA helix.

XXI. The Leper

~~Forsake me not, O Lord: O my God, be not far from me.~~
Psalm 38:21

The poor leper. The lowly leper. The cursed leper. The "run away"--- leper!

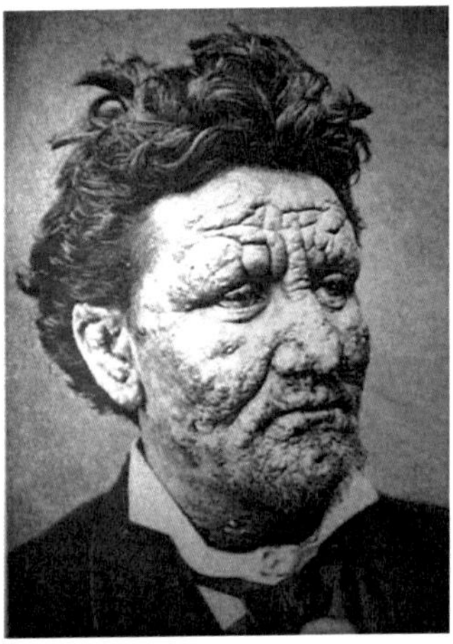
The poor leper.

Throughout the Bible, the leper is a diseased person who may be healed by the High Priests, as seen in Leviticus. Jesus in an interesting story cures ten lepers in just one of many examples of His healing powers. Yet only one of the ten actually thanks Him! Jesus recognizes the lack of gratitude of the "nine," but does not comment further, rather focusing his blessing on the one man, a Samaritan, who gave thanks (31); I found at least 22 separate references to lepers in the Bible, so it must be an important disease to God.

The fact that leprosy is still a tremendous health problem in the world should not surprise us. India and Brazil have the most cases, with many millions infected with this bacteria (or more specifically mycobacterium, in the same general category as tuberculosis). When I was in medical school at the University of Miami, we rotated through the dermatology department, and there is actually a separate leprosy clinic at Jackson Memorial Hospital, where we treated patients, most of whom were originally from South America. All I ever knew about leprosy until then was from Monty Python and the movie Papillon!

I still don't know much about this disease, nor have I seen a case since, but that doesn't really matter, for as you'll discover truth is stranger than fiction.

Start with another name for leprosy, Hansen's disease, an eponym for the Norwegian doctor who first isolated the

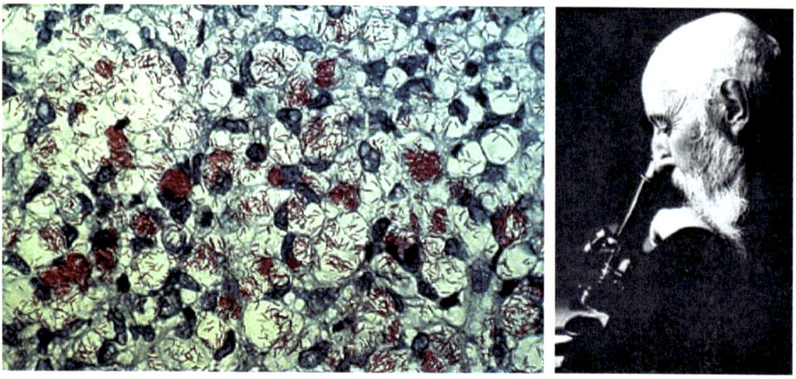

Dr. Hansen and the bacterium that still infects millions of people in the world.

bacillus in 1873. This was early in the history of bacteriology, and to identify a causative agent of any sort was huge. But not much happened for nearly 70 years, when antibiotics were found tobe modestly effective in controlling this disease. As antibiotics were developed they were tested on patients, and with better treatments, sometimes, a side effect was observed. This side effect was the result of massive death of the mycobacterium in the skin, which caused another type of skin reaction called erythema nodosum leprosum. This was extremely painful and in desperation an Israeli physician named Jacob Sheskin found some bottles of thalidomide lying around and (don't ask me why), he tried the pills on a patient and his condition improved. Then Dr. Sheskin tried it on more people, and they also improved. In fact nearly every one with erythema nodosum leprosum treated with thalidomide got better!

Created by chemists at a small pharmaceutical company, in Germany, thalidomide was in every other respect a disaster of unspeakable proportions. It was originally synthesized in an attempt to create a new type of antibiotic, but in tests it had no activity in experimental animals. Since it was well tolerated, and rather than throw it out, the scientists convinced themselves that it might be useful as a sedative. So they gave free samples to physicians and eventually it was believed to be a nontoxic therapy for pregnant women with morning sickness.

No tests in pregnant animals were done but that didn't stop clinicians and scientists to agree that thalidomide was safe,

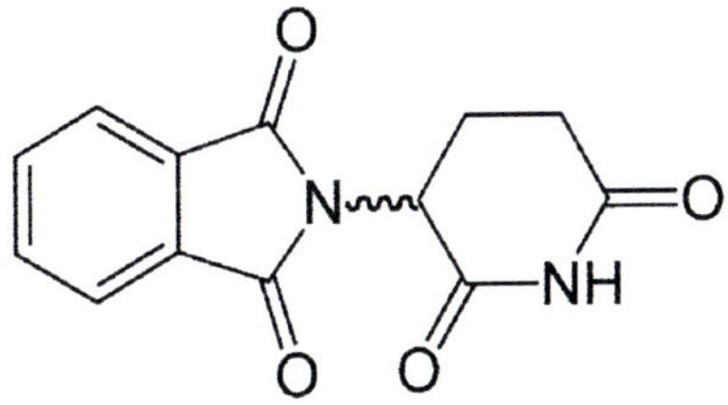

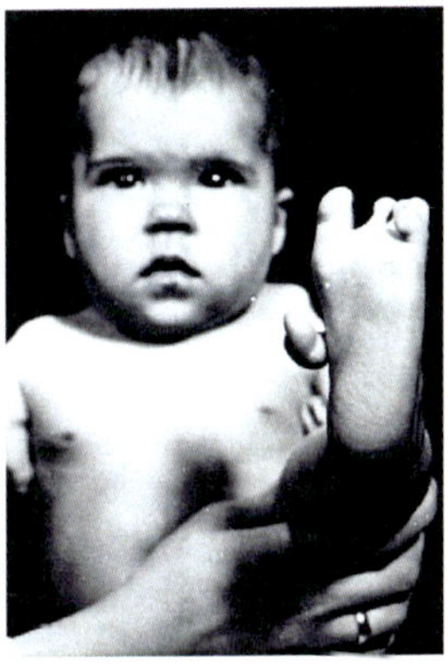

Structure of thalidomide and the terrible consequences of its improper use.

so in treating newly (1st trimester) pregnant women a horrible consequence was the eventual delivery of babies with phocomelia, where their limbs were grossly malformed, sort of in a flipper shape. So-called thalidomide babies were the result of a poorly conceived, improperly tested, ineffective and dangerous drug, which led to major changes in the way future drugs would be tested and approved. It was a terrible learning experience.

In trying to figure out the mechanism of action of thalidomide as a teratogen, scientists found that it inhibited blood vessel development (angiogenesis) in the developing embryo and fetus. In the early 1970's, the theory that tumors needed to create their own blood vessels to grow was advocated by Dr. Judah Folkman and his colleagues, so the next question was whether thalidomide might be effective in shrinking cancers.

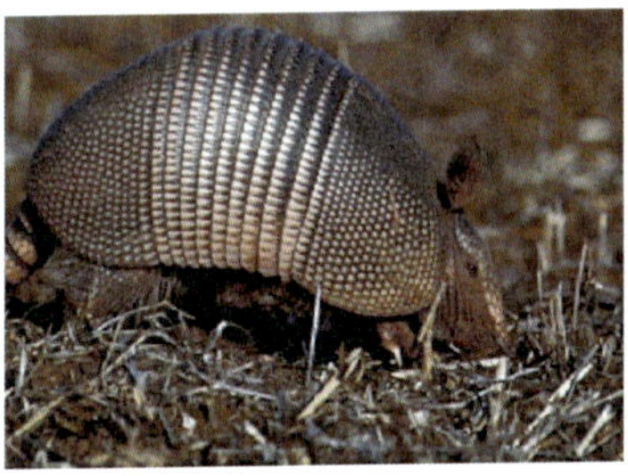

No one would believe the armadillo's usefulness in leprosy research if it weren't true!

Before we pursue that question, consider that for nearly 100 years after its discovery, no one could grow mycobacterium leprae in culture medium. While all these other events were unraveling, many millions of people were still being infected. Then in 1974 Dr. Eleanor Storrs reported on the isolation of the leprosy bug from armadillos! (32) And so to a large extent we owe much of what we have learned about leprosy from, of all creatures, the armadillo, which looks to me like an armor plated rat.

With further studies on thalidomide it appeared that it could decrease inflammatory responses, decrease angiogenesis, and paradoxically activate immune cells, in biochemical processes that are still not fully understood. But why would that stop anyone from testing this drug on nonpregnant patients with cancer, for in desperation, people will try just about anything?

In 1999, a year after the FDA approved thalidomide for treating an occasional complication of leprosy treatment, Dr. Bart Barlogie (one of the leading experts in myeloma), reported it to be effective in some patients with a hematologic malignancy called multiple myeloma. In combination with another drug called dexamethasone (which is a steroid drug that typically inhibits allergic reactions and immune function), thalidomide became a star chemotherapy drug in a Rube Goldberg series of scientific events. Newer thalidomide derivatives work even better, such as Revlimid, and all I can say is you can't make this stuff up!

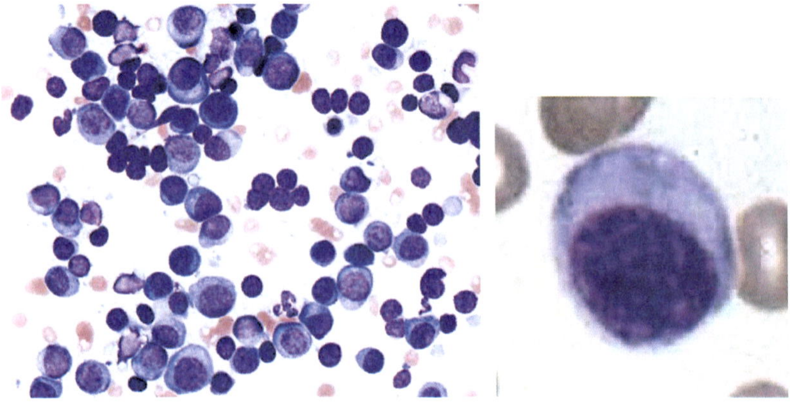

Myeloma cells as seen in the inset can be treated with a most peculiar drug regimen.

So:
Leper + horrible drug + Dr. Hansen + armadillo + desperation = myeloma therapy.

XXII. For Whom the Bell Curve Tolls

~~Every man's life ends the same way. It is only the details of how he lived and how he died that distinguish one man from another.~~

Ernest Hemingway (1899-1961)

We are all dots on the bell curve of life.

If you know about geometry, algebra, differential equations, probability theory*, and calculus, please read this with caution and pity. I really don't remember any "higher" mathematics, having forgotten nearly all of it. But, I know enough about the bell curve (or any other distribution of data points in a curve-like graph) to write this essay.

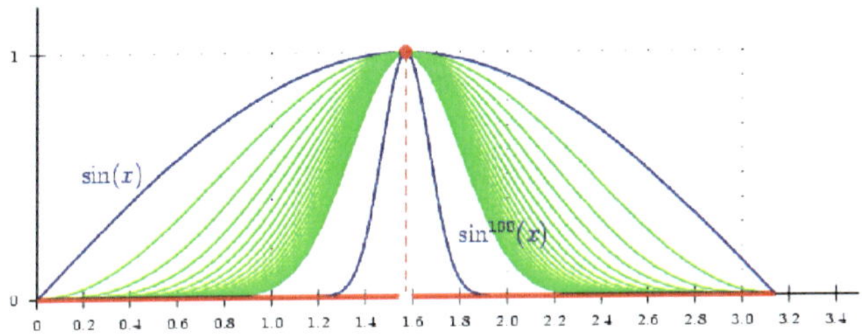

We are all dots on the bell curve of life.

When we talk about response rates for cancer patients, as I've mentioned before, we are talking about the measurement of something. In a typical study, drug A may shrink a tumor by more than 50%, for at least one month, in let's say 30% of people with a particular type of cancer. If we consider this simple example, then we would conclude that the response rate for drug A (a major response based on more than 50% of the tumor disappearing), is 30%, so if we treat 1,000 people with cancer, 300 will be expected to have a major response, assuming a similar age, performance status, stage of disease, and other comorbidities.

Now we can plot these responses on a graph, which may start to look like a bell curve, after we're done with this exercise.

* **As mentioned earlier, the genius of Blaise Pascal was not restricted to my earlier descriptions of his famous "wager." He was also the creator of probability theory.**

Each person among the 1,000 becomes a dot (or data point) on the graph of responses to drug A.

Now, let's add to the complexity, by including the other 700 people (dots), who represent the majority of other responses (or lack thereof). Let's say, another 300 patients have a minor response where their tumor shrinks in size by less than 50% but more than 25%. Add them to the curve. Now let's say another 300 patients have a reduction in size of their tumor, somewhere between less than 25% and not at all. This is typically called stable disease. Add them to the curve. And let's say another 100 (now the total is 1,000), have their tumor continue to grow in size by more than 25% while being treated (anything less than 25% growth is still considered stable disease by convention), then that is called disease progression. And add them too.

What about the people with major responses? Some may even see their tumor completely disappear, which we call a complete response. Or other responses of a similar magnitude (90% shrinkage for example), called near-complete responses. And so on ad infinitum (or nearly so).

Congratulations! You are a budding cancer statistician. And as a thought experiment, try to imagine all the possible variations we could graph in this study.

Consider the example of patient 997, enrolled to receive experimental drug A. Let's call him by a secret code word to protect his identity. How about patient 997=Buddy (all Buddy's of the world, please forgive me).

Buddy receives drug A for 3 weeks, with the fourth week off to rest from the toxic effects of drug A (we can graph that too). He has a CT scan before treatment, and at one month, read by a radiologist, who measures the size of the tumor before and after treatment. The radiologist calculates that the index tumor (the one he is comparing, and not any other tumors that may also be present), which was 2.0 cm (a little less than an inch) in greatest dimension, has now decreased in size to 1.1 cm.

So Buddy returns to the clinic and sees the oncologist to discuss his test results. Buddy is a nervous guy to begin with, so when the oncologist walks into the exam room, Buddy is standing, having read everything, and pacing back and forth, waiting at least ten minutes, with tremendous trepidation, and

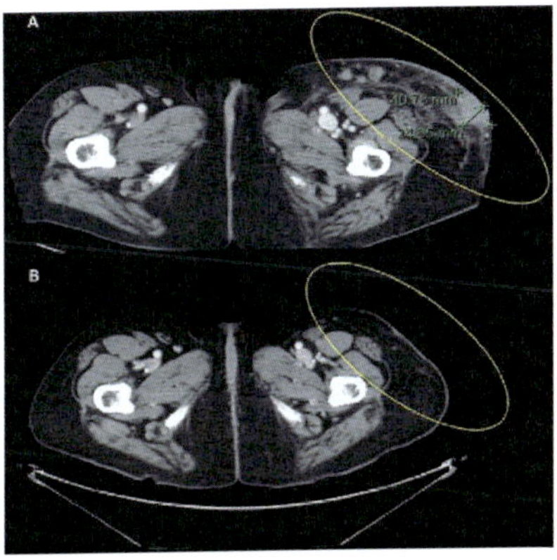

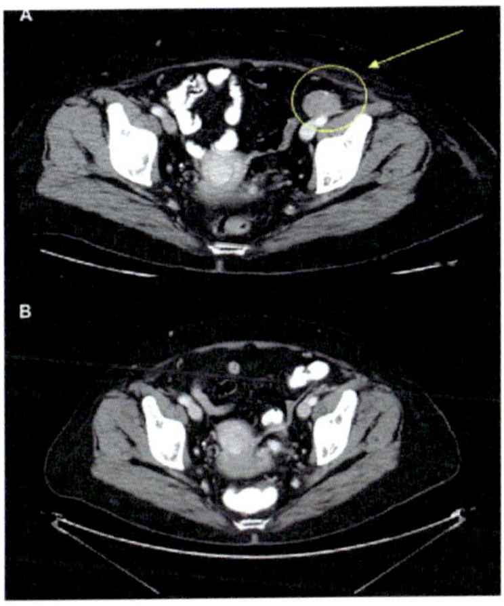

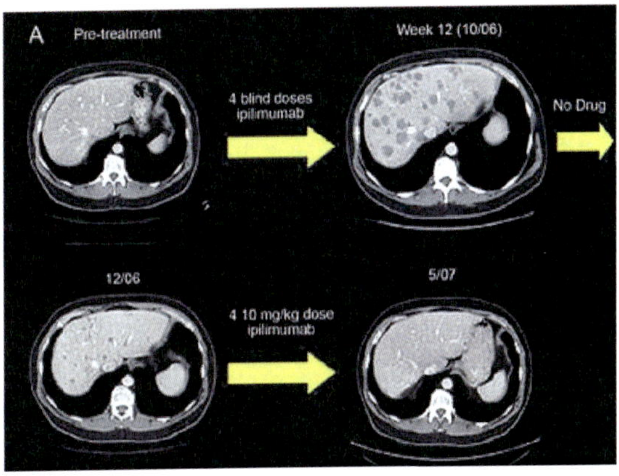

Beautiful examples of radiologic responses to therapy (in this case an experimental monoclonal antibody). But this is only part of the story.

Buddy says: "Hi Doc, What about the scan?"

Now if you were the oncologist what would you say?*

a) "Before I tell you the results of your CT scan, I need to ask you some questions, as part of the clinical trial, and then examine you, and then we'll talk about the CT scan results."

*** In a new book by the prolific Christian author, Walter Wangerin, Jr., *"Letters From The Land of Cancer"*, he uses the term "chemical oncologists" to distinguish them from the "radiation oncologists", to describe the medical oncologists treating him for advanced lung cancer.**

b) "What scan results?"
c) "Buddy, be cool."
d) "The scan shows a minor response to drug A."
e) "The scan shows nearly a major response to drug A."
f) "Not bad, Buddy, not bad at all."
g) "Pretty good, Buddy, pretty good."
h) "Sit down."
i) "Buddy, how are you feeling, are you feeling lucky today?"

Beyond a point on the bell curve (or whatever curve) of response rates, have we accomplished anything real or tangible? For the cancer may have decreased in size anyway by other mechanisms. Or the cancer may have decreased in size, but the remaining cells, (some of which may be so-called cancer stem cells) (33), may be intrinsically resistant to drug A, and they have already spread to other, as yet undetected sites. Or Buddy is experiencing unacceptable toxicity from drug A, despite a potentially meaningful response, and must be removed from the study, as part of the protocol. Or he feels great and is ecstatic about the CT results....

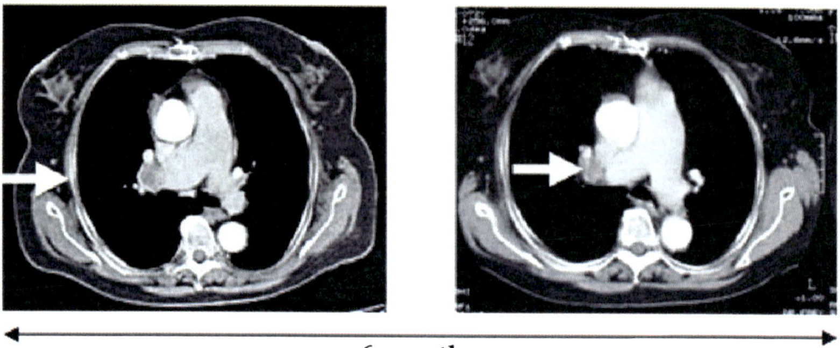

6 months

Sometimes stable disease is a perfectly desirable outcome.

Or how about drug A delaying the time to disease progression, but not changing the survival rate. An example of this type of outcome was recently reported in the news that led to the rejection of Avastin for metastatic breast cancer (34) (and yes men get breast cancer, although I don't think Buddy would be eligible for participation), by an FDA advisory panel by a

5-to-4 vote. (I'll bet it will be approved, with more data, having already been approved in Europe).*

Buddy wants to know one thing: is drug A working? In his way of thinking, which is all too common, shrinking the size of the cancer equals drug A working. But, this is incorrect reasoning for what Buddy really wants to know, as I suppose most of us do, is: "Is drug A going to significantly prolong my life, with a modest and manageable toxicity, or not?" And the answer to that question is, of course: "I don't know."

For what does it mean when a tumor decreases in size for a period of time? Are we really expected to believe that changing the size of a quarter size spot to a nickel size spot on a CT scan is a reflection of our capacity to survive for long periods of time with advanced cancer?

I believe that beyond the reductionist's need to "place that dot," the answers to these important questions will come from scientists and clinicians, of great courage and intellectual curiosity, stepping back and reflecting on what we are ignoring in these studies. One point (pun intended) to consider, that is rarely mentioned or measured, in the bell curve of cancer life, is what role drug A has (in perhaps unexpected and even paradoxical ways), in influencing the immune response to cancer, which may be the "sleeping tiger" in much of what we observe and attribute to other etiologies in cancer research.

*** FDA approval was finally given, despite the advisory panel's objections.**

XXIII. How Should Cancer Patients Respond to Response Rates?

~~"The saddest aspect of life right now is that science gathers knowledge faster than society gathers wisdom."~~ Isaac Asimov (1920-1992)

One of the fascinating features of cancer is that people can go to their doctor complaining of some fairly mild and non-descript symptoms such as feeling more tired and end up with a diagnosis of widespread, i.e., metastatic cancer.

After completing what is called a staging workup with CT, PET/CT, MRI, and other radiologic tests, along with routine laboratory studies, I have seen countless patients with an incredible amount of disease and yet few signs or symptoms. And remember that the cancer was probably present for years before being discovered.

So the first question is: How can people walk around with a considerable disease burden and not know it?

The second question is: How important is it to make the cancer partially or completely disappear for a period of time?

The third question is: If the cancer disappears will the patient feel better and live longer?

As we have talked about before, when oncologists talk about cancer disappearing, what they are really talking about is something called a response rate. This is the percentage of patients who have disease (that can be measured by some method such as size of a mass on a CT scan), that shrinks down to a smaller size or disappears completely. There are also laboratory tests that sometimes are used to measure biochemical responses in a similar fashion.

The precise definition of a complete radiologic response is the complete disappearance of measurable disease for at least one month. After one month if the cancer grows back, we don't change our definition that a complete response was achieved.

In a similar fashion, a partial response indicates the cancer decreased in size by more than 25%.

No response actually means the cancer decreased in size by less than 25% or not at all, although sometimes one hears about something called a minor response in this setting.*

To complicate matters further, a major response can be described, as indicating that the cancer decreased in size by more than 50%, but not completely.

To really make you dizzy, there are also mixed responses where the cancer may shrink in some places but remain the same size or increase in other places.

Let us not ignore other terms such as complete remission and cytogenetic remission, which are typically used to describe blood diseases such as myeloma, lymphoma, and leukemia.

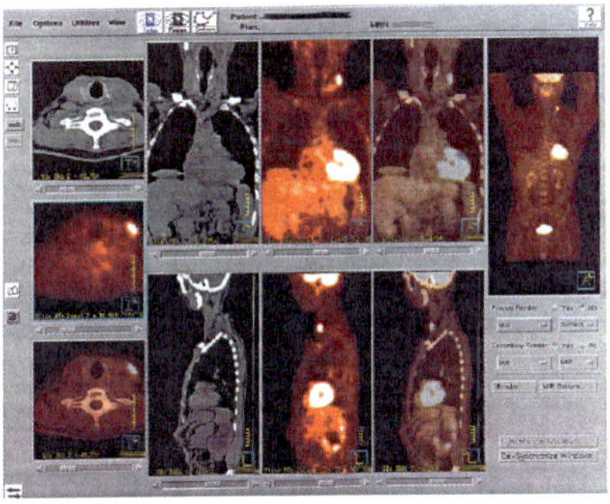

PET/CT scans of a patient with a malignant tumor in the left neck (the heart ahd brain normally are hyper-metabolic). What does it truly tell us?

To add to our confusion, a patient can have a biochemical response such as a decrease in PSA, CEA, CA27.29, CA15-3, CA19-9, CA 125... and yet the CT scans or other radiologic tests show no change!

And with new tests such as PET/CT, which measure the metabolic activity of cancer and its size and distribution, we can sometimes observe a metabolic response where the tumor seems to have shut down its excessive utilization of glucose (or other substrates) and yet its size is unchanged.

So when is a response not a response? The answer depends on what we are really talking about and part of that discussion is based on concepts such as quality of life and prolonged survival, which may not be improved with cancer treatments that demonstrate statistically significant response rates.

So a word of caution: Do not always equate response rates with feeling better and living longer!

* **The precise definition of response rates including different measurement standards is continually changing.**

XXIV. Has Reefer Madness Struck the National Cancer Institute?

~~"I don't do drugs. I am drugs."~~ Salvador Dali (1904-1989)

Not too long ago, a patient told me she watched a news clip describing the possible use of marijuana in treating cancer. I was reluctant to investigate further but within a few days reports started to surface about a study published in the Journal of the National Cancer Institute describing the anticancer effect of a marijuana derivative that has been used (legally) in treating patients who experience side effects from chemotherapy drugs such as nausea and vomiting.

This drug is called Marinol and it is a synthetic version of tetrahydrocannabinol (THC), which is one of the active chemicals in pot plants (Cannabis sativa in our country).

Before you tell your friends and family that getting high has unexpected benefits in treating metastatic cancer, read on.

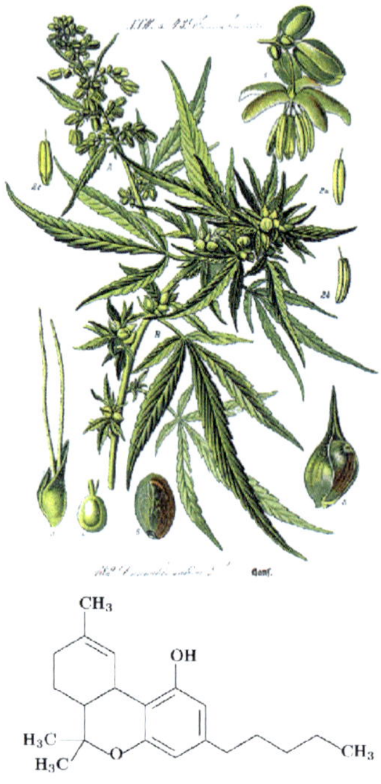

Cannabis and THC: Plant and psychoactive substance.

The study by Ramer and Hinz (35) uses cancer cells which grow outside of the body. These are called tissue culture cells. There many hundreds of cell lines derived from animals and humans with cancer which have been adapted to grow outside of a host, and these cell lines can be studied biochemically to determine how they are affected by altering their environment. One way to do this is to add chemicals to these cells and see what happens. When we talk about in vitro experiments (versus in vivo) this is what we are talking about. Any potential effect observed in vitro, such as the death of cancer cells by adding chemical X, must be confirmed by observations in vivo (i.e., in a living creature), before we can even begin to ask questions like: Does drug X help patients with cancer in any meaningful way?*

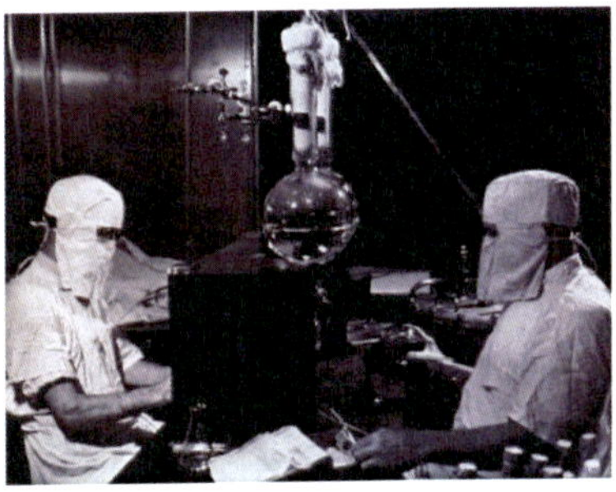

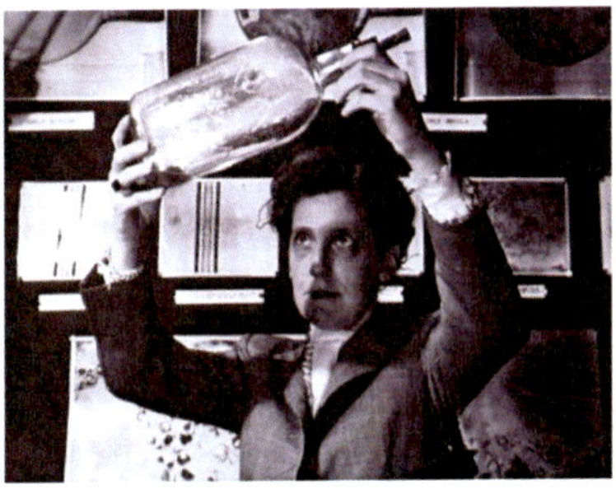

Give me that old-time tissue culture.

In this study one of the chemicals was THC. THC was structurally characterized in 1964. THC will get you high. THC will make you forget what I just said. THC will make you want to check the refrigerator right now for snacks. But I doubt THC will ever be used to control metastatic cancer.

THC and other cannabinoids derived from pot binds to receptors in the brain that influence neurological and psychological function, and these receptors are called CB1. There are also CB2 receptors found in other cell types such as spleen cells of the immune system. THC also affects other cells, and their functions, probably by binding to other receptors. So in treating cancer cells with THC, Ramer and Hinz showed that certain cell lines could be inhibited from becoming invasive in an in vitro assay using a gel matrix to measure invasiveness. This process was mediated by another molecule produced by these cells called TIMP-1 (Tissue Inhibitor of Matrix Metalloproteinase-1). Matrix metalloproteinases may be a key molecule in the spread of cancer cells as they help break apart the natural barriers that prevent cancer cells from growing and spreading. THC somehow promotes the expression of TIMP-1.

In 1975 a paper was published in the (guess) Journal of the National Cancer Institute titled: "Anticancer Activity of Cannabinoids."(35) This study in mice demonstrated that THC

*** These are called pre-clinical studies.**

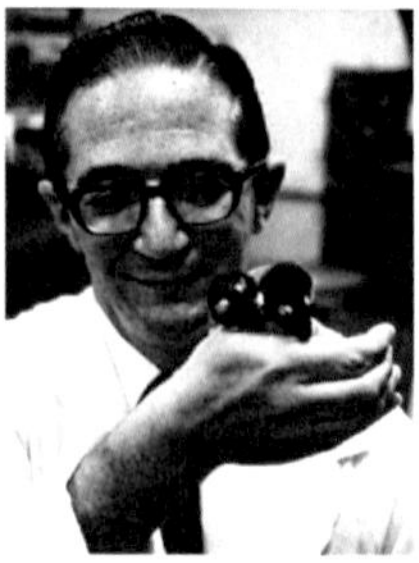

Happy investigator. Why?

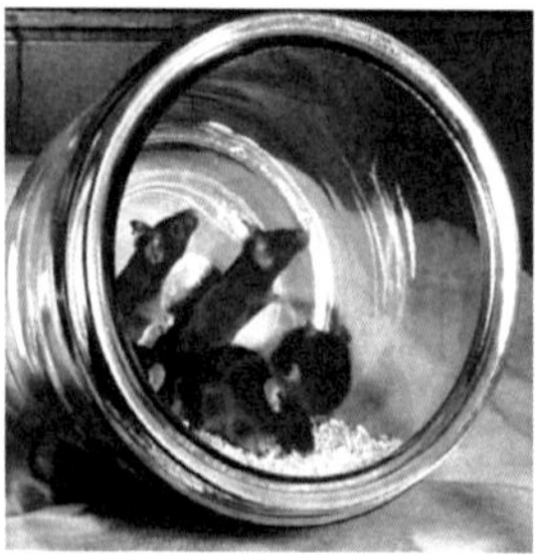

Mice ready to party!

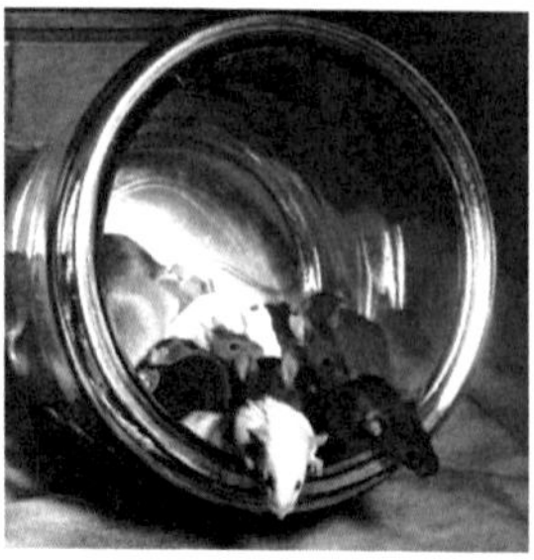

Party over!

could inhibit lung cancer growth in vivo and in vitro by feeding mice THC every day for nearly 2 weeks. Other types of cancer cells were also studied. But beyond creating incredibly stoned mice*, the results were less than spectacular.

Fast forwarding 30 years we are back where we started in that THC is being studied by researchers (including clinical trials in humans with advanced brain cancers), (36) lung cancer where it seems to have an anticancer effect, (37) lung cancer where it seems to promote cancer growth, (38) and many other cancer cell types with contradictory results.

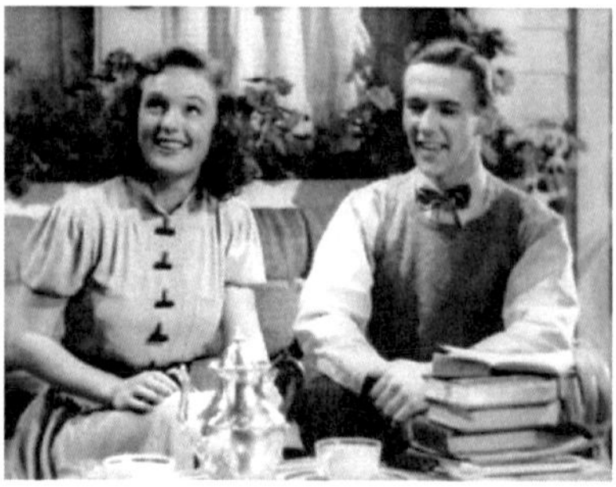

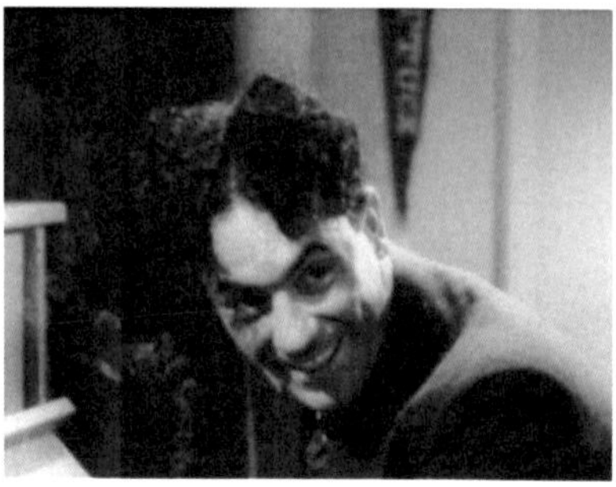

Scenes from the original movie Reefer Madness. No wonder they are smiling.

My opinion is that the use of THC and other related molecules in treating cancer, as a form of chemotherapy, will fail. THC is wonderful in altering perception but not wonderful in decreasing cancer invasiveness. And as for the news media treating what I consider a mediocre paper as something sent

*** The use of marijuana as a "recreational" drug in humans, and its consequences, is a political, social and medical nightmare.**

from heaven, a quote to leave you with from the great skeptic Mark Twain: "A lie can travel halfway around the world while the truth is putting on its shoes."

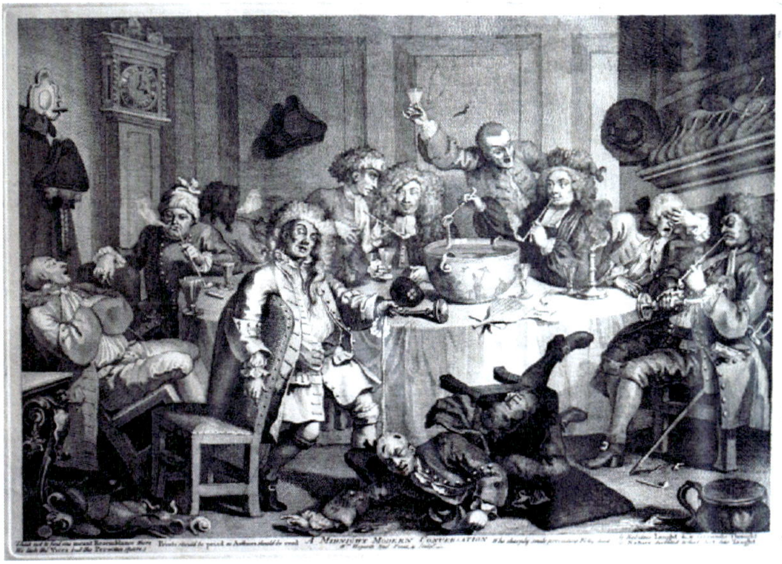

Author's conception of the article review board of the Journal of the National Cancer Institute.

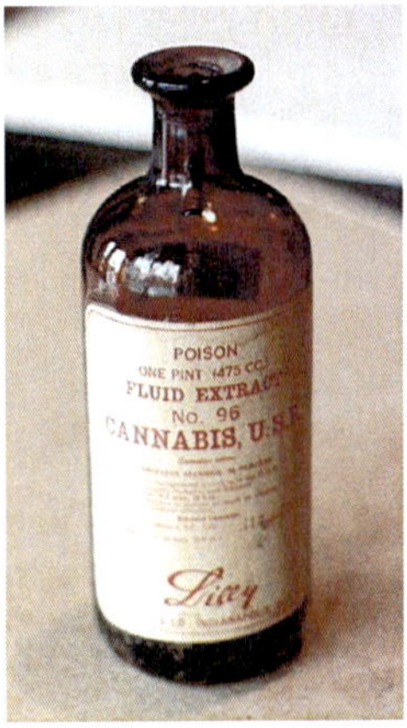

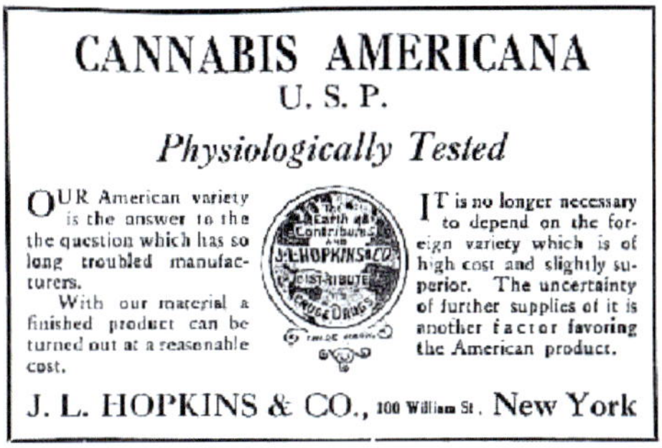

Early 1900's marketing of cannabis extract.

XXV. Phraseotics

~~"When one door closes, another opens; but we often look so long and so regretfully upon the closed door that we do not see the one which has opened for us."~~ Alexander Graham Bell (1847-1922)

I have to admit that I suffer from a condition which I just invented named for Alexander Graham Bell*, the man who transformed communications, by developing and marketing the telephone. The telephone and its subsequent offspring, the cellular phone, are communication tools that allow us to speak to each other at pretty much anytime and anywhere. When I think about our ability to translate electrical impulses into recognizable aural signals which the brain can process and understand, it is nothing short of amazing. To do this at distances of thousands of miles, without paper cups and string, allowing for irregularities in transmission ("you're cutting out"), encourages me that we may survive and advance as a species.

As to the definition of this disease: "A condition where words are spoken, but not always completely understood." Please see the theory of Selective Hearing.

Now the theory of Selective Hearing*, which I just invented, is that, unlike computers, the human brain is capable

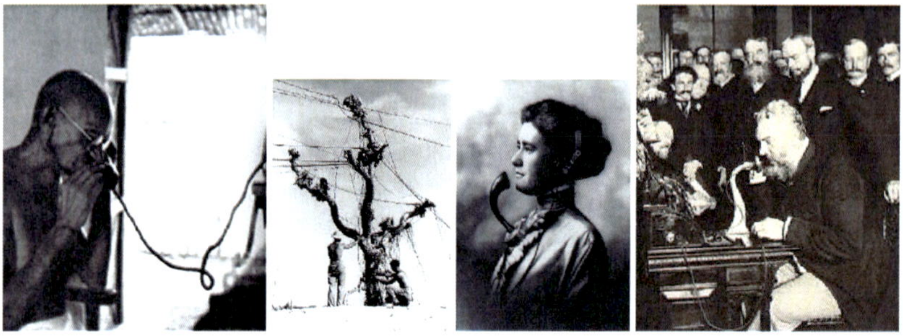

Author's imaginary conversation between Gandhi and Alexander Graham Bell.

*** I am not sure what to call it. The eponym "Alexander" disease which I planned to use is already taken. This disease is a genetic disease that causes infants and children to develop terrible neurological problems of all sorts. There is an adult onset form as well. "Alexander Disease," J Rafael Gorospe, MD, PhD in Gene Reviews, National Center for Biotechnology Information (NCBI) website.**

of the most incredibly dumb conclusions, after processing the simplest statements.

For example, as in the game "telephone," which I suspect is no longer a popular game for teens, start out with a phrase or statement, lets say: "The surgeon said he got it all, so I'm not sure why I'm seeing an oncologist." After ten or so "phone calls," the message is transformed by some incredibly sophisticated neural network into: "The oncologist said I may die."

After many thousands of patient encounters, here is one synthetic scenario, or as physicians like to say, "clinical vignette."

A 68-year-old man with recently resected stage IIIA colon cancer is seen in initial consultation two weeks after surgery. He is a captain of industry, a multimillionaire who owns a manufacturing company, with several hundred employees. He is recovering well after surgery, with no unusual complaints. His other relevant medical problems include coronary artery disease, with a heart attack at age 54, and subsequent angioplasty and stent placement at age 62. Other than heart and blood pressure medicines (and Viagra), and mild diabetes and arthritis, he takes no other drugs, including no vitamins or supplements.**

In my careful review of the pathology report (which is probably the most important thing that I do), the tumor was located in the transverse colon, measuring about 5 cm in greatest diameter (which is not relevant to staging or prognosis), with the histological description typical for this type of malignancy, "a moderately differentiated adenocarcinoma, with tumor extending into the muscularis propria of the bowel wall, but not through it. All resection margins were clear, with the closest margin 1 cm (distal margin). A total of 18 mesenteric lymph nodes were identified, of which 3 were positive for metastatic disease; formal pathologic staging is therefore pT2pN1Mx."

** **Unless specifically stated, all clinical scenarios were modified to protect my patients' privacy.**

Prior to surgery, this mover and shaker, waited about 6 months before seeing his internist, and reporting occasional bloody stools (he was hoping it was just hemorrhoids), but within a week, all the necessary tests (CT scan, colonoscopy with biopsy, preop lab tests including CEA and CA19-9, cardiology consult) were completed.

The CT scan of the abdomen and pelvis showed a mass in the transverse colon, and no clear evidence of lymph node involvement or spread to other sites, such as the liver. Despite smoking from age 20 to 50, a CT of the chest was not included in the preop radiological studies (the lung bases were mentioned as being clear on the abdominal CT report). All chemistries (including liver function tests and LDH--lactate dehydrogenase) and CBC (complete blood count) were normal. Tumor markers (including PSA, ordered by me) were either normal or just slightly above normal (CEA was 4.0, which in nonsmokers was abnormal, with 2.5 considered the upper limit of normal, and the other markers were within the range of normal).

So how does the statement: "The surgeon said he got it all, so why am I seeing an oncologist?" become: "He said I may die."

Let's dissect these statements from the patient's perspective or cancer gestalt:

1) He got it all: Translation: All the cancer was removed, so I'm cured. If they can't see any disease on the scans and the lab tests are OK, then there is no cancer remaining, and therefore I'm cured. Please tell me I'm cured.

2) Why am I seeing an oncologist? Translation: I denied my symptoms for several months, even though I knew bloody stools could be cancer. I don't want to die of cancer. This is just a bad dream. If I close my eyes, everything will be perfect again.

Now the same analysis from the oncologist's viewpoint:

1) He got it all: Translation: I'm sure the surgeon (who I know well, and is seasoned and careful with his language) didn't just say that; he probably said something like: "The operation was successful, all the cancer was removed that

the pathologist could see, but since there were lymph nodes with cancer, I want you to talk to an oncologist, who may recommend chemotherapy."

2) Why am I seeing an oncologist?: Translation: I understand you don't want to deal with this difficult situation. You want reassurance that your life will return to normal, and the power and control which have shaped your career can continue to be used in this situation as well. By sheer force of will, you will make the oncologist and any treatment he recommends irrelevant.

The emotive content of events supersedes any rational evaluation that may occur. Or as the philosopher Anonymous (I guess he was Greek) once said: "People hear what they want to hear. People believe what they want to believe. And in the never-ending internal dialogue between the irrational and the rational, who do you think is going to win?"

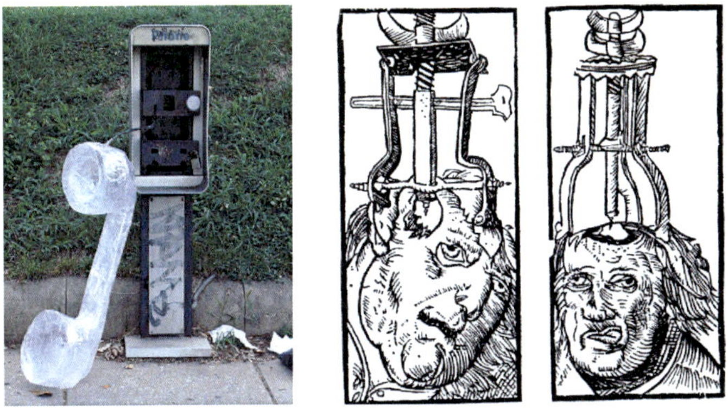

Author's impressions after playing the "cancer telephone game."

Hence the newest linguistic creation of mine, "phraseotics," which I just defined in the previous paragraph. So when you ask your spouse something, don't expect the answer or response you had hoped for, the same with your kids, coworkers, and pretty much anyone you speak to.

But do not despair, for your dog understands you perfectly (cats are another story)!

As for the end of this story, create your own, I'm taking my dogs for a nice long hike.

XXVI. The Age of Age

~~Death be not proud, though some have called thee Mighty and dreadful, for, thou art not so, For, those, whom thou think'st, thou dost overthrow, Die not, poore death, nor yet canst thou kill me.~~ John Donne (1572-1631)

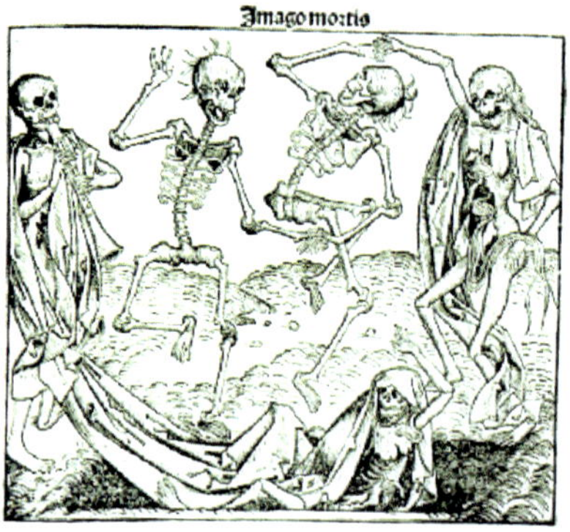

A 15th Century image of Death hooting it up.

People are living longer. In developed countries such as the United States, the life expectancy is nearly 80 years, and there is no reason it cannot continue to increase. I'm not sure what the theoretical limit is for humans, but figure around 120 is about it, and then one passes on to another state of being called death.*

From a biblical perspective, early on people lived to extraordinary, tree-like ages. For instance, Methuselah is the oldest lived human at 969 years, and others, including Noah, lived well into the 800's. Moses only made it to 120, but his age and manner of death (taken by

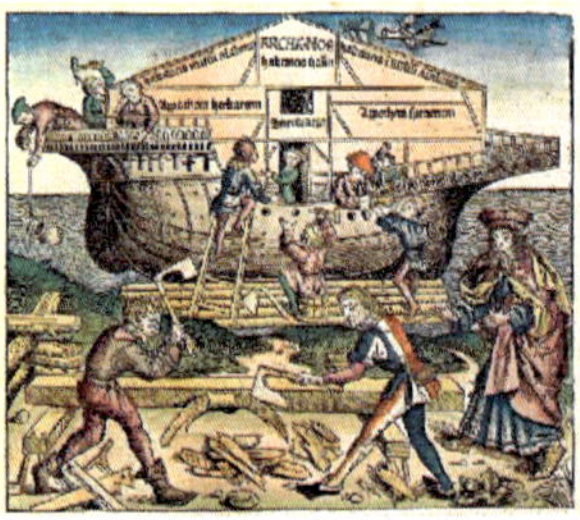

Nuremberg chronicles.

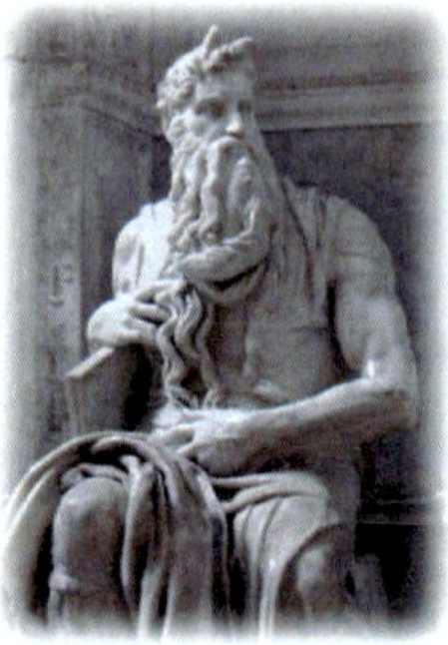

Michelangelo's "Moses"

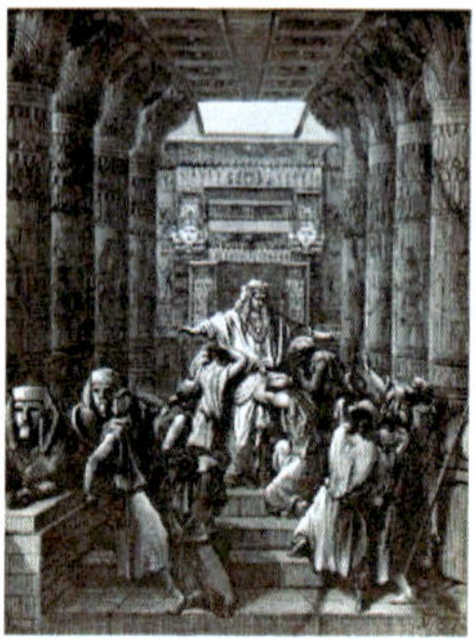

Dore's interpretation of the bibilical scene: Joseph makes himself known to his brethren.

Biblical Old-Timers: Noah kept busy. Moses kept moving. Joseph kept getting in trouble.

*** The US government publishes actuarial tables on life expectancy. It stops at age 119!**

God still pretty spry), has for many religious people remained the gold standard for longevity. Less prominent figures like you and I may expect 80 to be considered a righteous age to pass on, for a righteous life led.

But living longer may not be living better. Some people end up with debilitating diseases that impair their ability to function independently. Their families, despite their best efforts cannot take care of them, so they end up in nursing homes, where many become so disillusioned, they just wait to die.

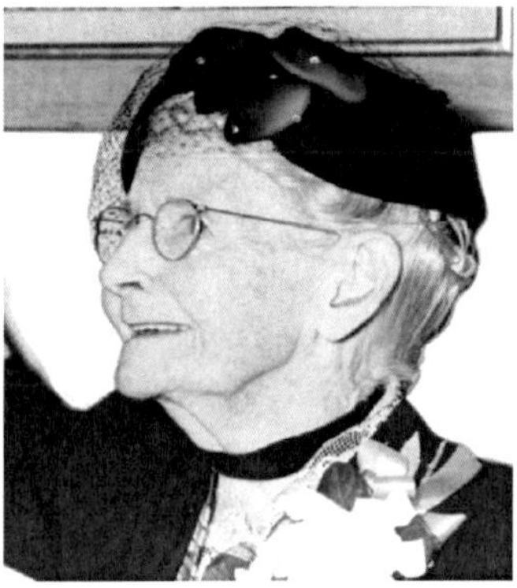

The late-blooming painter, Grandma Moses (1860-1961). As my late Grandpa Benny* said: "The first 100 years are the hardest."

Other people may be more highly functional, or motivated and fight on. Still, as I've experienced personally with my late father and now my mother, a nursing home is an imperfect but necessary solution to the problems associated with aging and disease.

Will the future of mankind be one in which people live so long that we will no longer be able to provide even a modicum of comfort, for most of its citizens? If you have enough money and/or really good insurance addressing long term care, this will not be a consideration, but most people struggle financially and don't have the resources to really plan adequately for the future. Nor can we entirely depend on government programs like Social Security, Medicare, or Medicaid to respond adequately to our aging population, as our nation is already running up an incredible debt. Other social and religious organizations may be able to help, but again the numbers are staggering.

I have no idea what to do about the "Age of Age," beyond the recommendation that people reconsider how old is old enough. For instance a friend of mine wants to live forever.

*** Grandpa Benny died at 97, so he was right!**

He says, "I want to be a raisin in a jar." I'm not kidding. He is an otherwise intelligent and fairly sensible person, but that's what he wants. A patient of mine with a terrible bile duct cancer that had already spread to his bones and other organs at the time of diagnosis, wanted everything done to sustain his life. He was already an amputee from end-stage diabetes and renal disease and had received a kidney transplant a couple years before, so he was not exactly the best candidate for aggressive treatment of any sort, but that is precisely what he believed would help him live many more years. His wife, who loved him dearly, told me she "wanted him to live for a thousand years." And she meant what she said. As an oncologist, I've heard many things, but I was taken aback by her completely irrational desires. The outcome, unfortunately, was more like a thousand hours of additional life with chemotherapy.

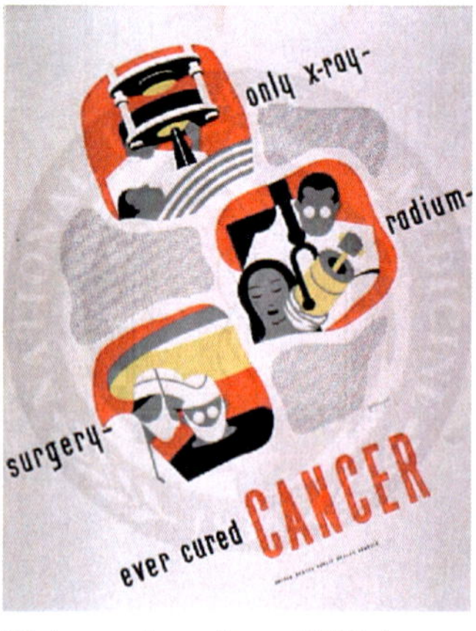

This poster, circa 1930, is no longer true. Advances made in treating cancer now allow us to "cure" people with chemotherapy and biological therapy, only to return with new cancers.

On the other hand, I've had people who were comfortable with death. One lady who was 79 and in a wheelchair, with a treatable and even potentially curable lymphoma, said: "I do not wish for any treatment that will prolong my life." Many other patients have also expressed similar views, which I deeply respect as a mature and sensible approach to terrible disease. No one need suffer beyond measure in these situations, and sometimes the treatment is toxic and ineffective and worse than the disease itself.

If you truly believe that cancer, in general, will be controlled with chemotherapy, radiation, surgery, or other treatments, I'm sorry to disappoint you. More and more people will develop cancer throughout the world as the global population increases and people live longer. Since the industrial revolution, (and I'm all for industry and technology), our planet has been drenched with toxic, carcinogenic chemicals, which we now know in the tiniest amounts, over say 20 to 60 years of chronic exposure, promote the development of a myriad of forms of cancer. If we just live long enough and wait, the likelihood is that we will develop cancer. That doesn't imply it can't be cured or controlled at times, but what I'm seeing more and more is a growing number of what I would call cancer "frequent flyers." I saw one woman with 5 different cancers who was still in very good shape at 75. And people with 3 separate malignancies are not unusual anymore.

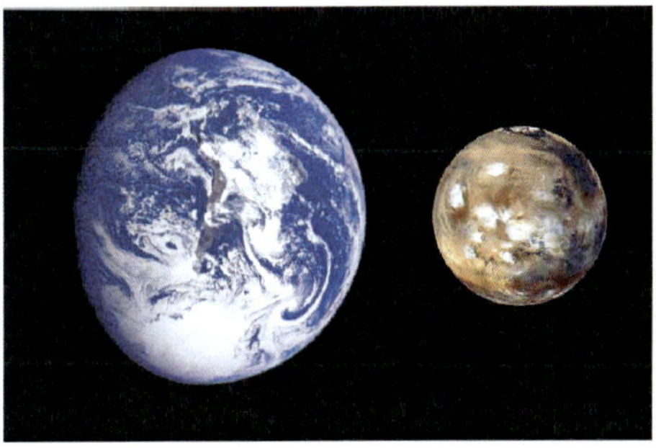

Toxic waste dump (Earth) and Mars. Don't expect any help from the Martians.

A healthy diet, exercise, prayer, vitamins, supplements, may help reduce the risk of cancer, or at least to delay its often inevitable development, but the hard numbers are that the benefits statistically are small, but significant. Small and significant does not equal control. For control to occur, we have to figure out how to prevent cancer by other more elegant methods. Decreasing pollution may help a little, but we already live in a toxic waste dump (planet Earth), which will take hundreds of years (if ever) to clean up. So I think it naive to think that "the cure" is something that can be achieved.

Now consider this equation: time + toxic chemicals (carcinogens) + viruses + genetic instability = cancer.

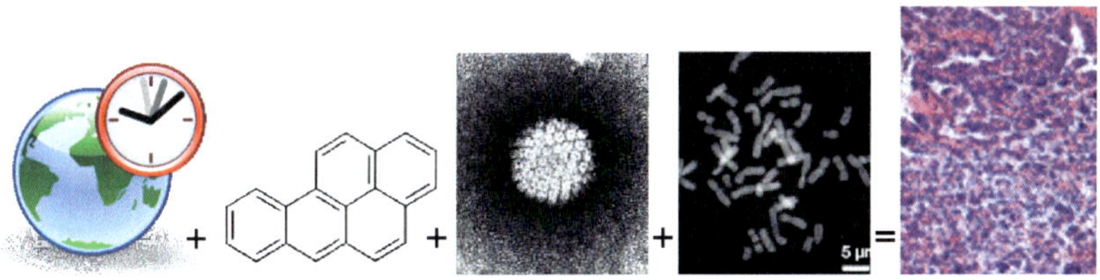

Visual aids for the equation above.

Time being time, is not fixed; so if we live long enough and don't die from something else (reader's choice), we'll probably develop cancer cells in our bodies. In fact, they're probably already there in all of us, every day. Remaining undetected for some of us, they are part of our genetic complexity. For cancer to become clinically apparent, the other factors in the equation may or may not need to be active. In other words, if you have a particularly dysfunctional genetic makeup like we see sometimes in cancer syndromes, you don't need anything else but time to develop cancer. In other cases, carcinogens or viruses alone are sufficient to trigger things. You get the idea, it's not that complicated!

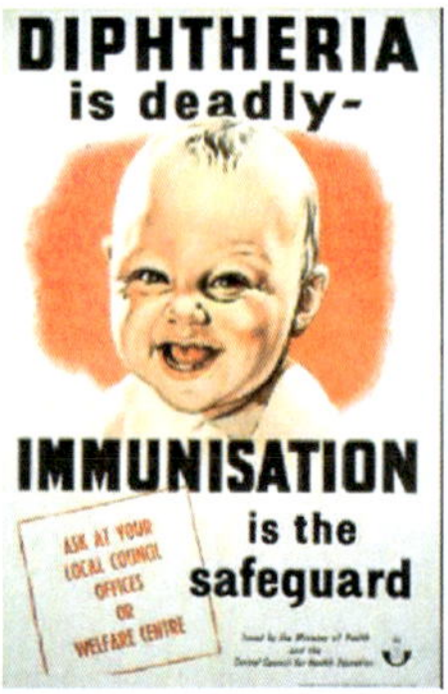

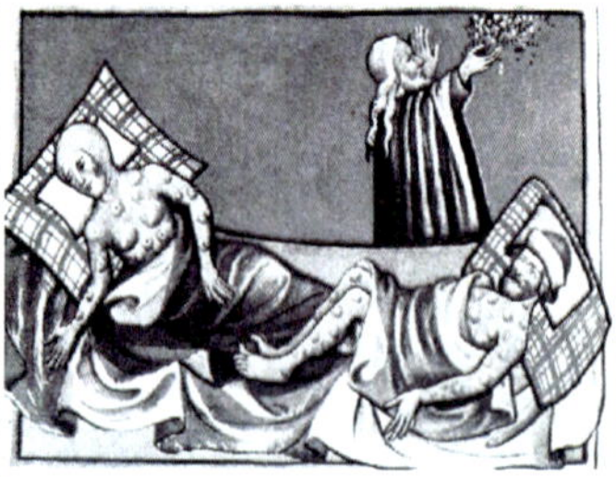

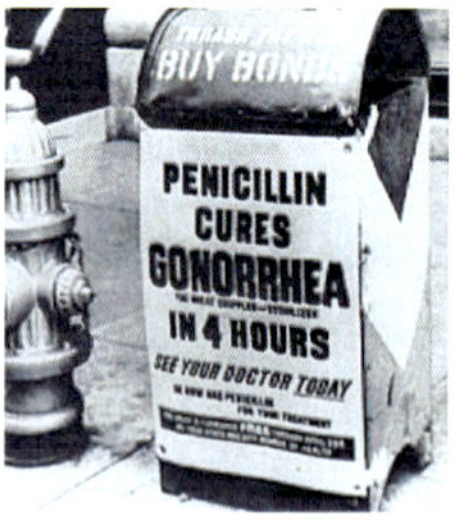

Before effective vaccines and antibiotics and other public health measures, an early death from infectious diseases was very common.

What are we to do? For let us not despair. The answer is to figure out a way to prevent cancer from ever occurring by creating very, very specific vaccines that help the good old immune system do its job more effectively. For the reason this is the "Age of Age" is to a large extent a consequence of improved public hygiene (less viruses and other bugs), vaccines to prevent or ameliorate infectious diseases and very, very specific molecules that kill microorganisms (antibiotics). Seventy five years ago people died from common infections, and now they are living much longer (statistically), so they can die from something else. Still, that something else need not be cancer. Cancer in many respects behaves like any other parasitic or infectious disease, only in a much more clever and sinister way, but to a large extent, I believe the principles are the same.

So then, how about the "Age of Age" transformed into the "Age of MAGE"? For MAGE is one of many molecules that the immune system (with an appropriate adjuvant), can become stimulated against and attack cancer cells, leading to

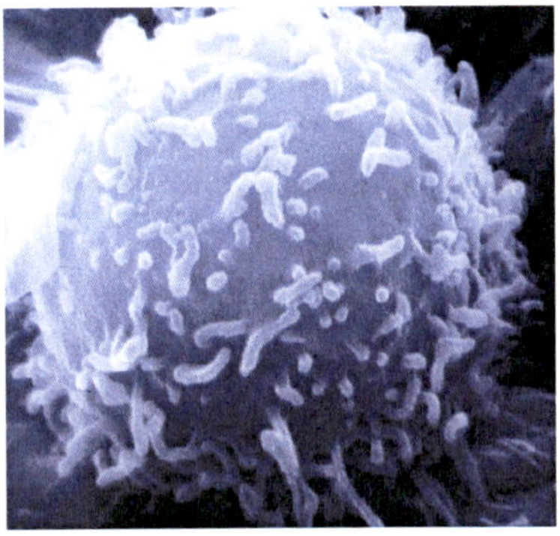

Regulating the powerful forces of the immune system, lymphocytes with various functions, are critical for cancer control.

their death, or at least inhibiting their growth. This is just the beginning of the "Age of MAGE," and other similar molecules which are displayed on cancer cells but not (with rare exception) any other normal cells. By creating immunogenic vaccines, we are treating cancer patients with early encouraging results.* In the future, similar vaccines may eventually be created that can prevent cancer from developing. In fact, I think the greatest advance in cancer immunotherapy in the 20th century was the development of the hepatitis B vaccine! Since liver cancer is often stimulated to develop by the hepatitis virus (B, C and such), vaccination against this virus seems to be having an incredible benefit in reducing the risk of cancer, by preventing infection from ever occurring.**

The Cancer Vaccine Collaborative is leading the way toward international efforts to control and maybe even prevent cancer in many millions of people throughout our planet, though we must not rush our conclusions. Scientific rigor and patience are really needed to do things correctly.

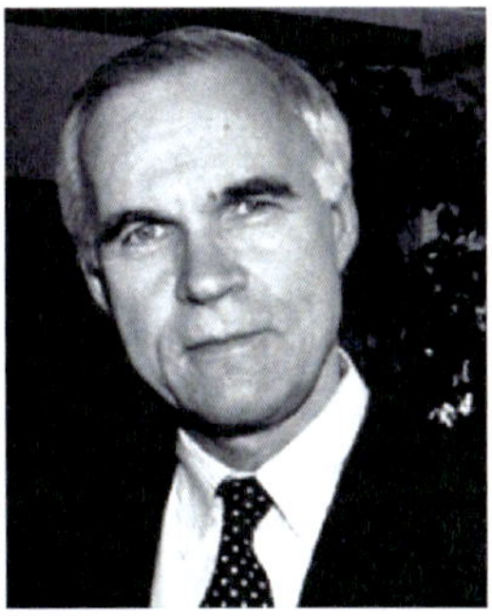

L.J. Old, MD, Founder of modern cancer immunology. c. 1988

I encourage you to access the Cancer Research Institute website and related linkages in the internet to learn more about these novel treatment strategies. And as you may have guessed, this approach is the brilliant creation of one man, Dr. Lloyd Old, who, as you know from earlier readings, is the founder of modern cancer immunology.

*** The MAGE-A3 vaccine made by GlaxoSmithKline is being studied intensely among cancer patients.**

**** A recent study from China showed that there was a 70% reduction in liver cancer in young people who were vaccinated about 20 years ago.**

XXVII. The Importance of Being Important

~~"Illusion is the first of all pleasures."~~ Oscar Wilde (1854-1900)

Look in the mirror; then return to your reading.

What did you see?

Did you see your self? Did you see your soul?

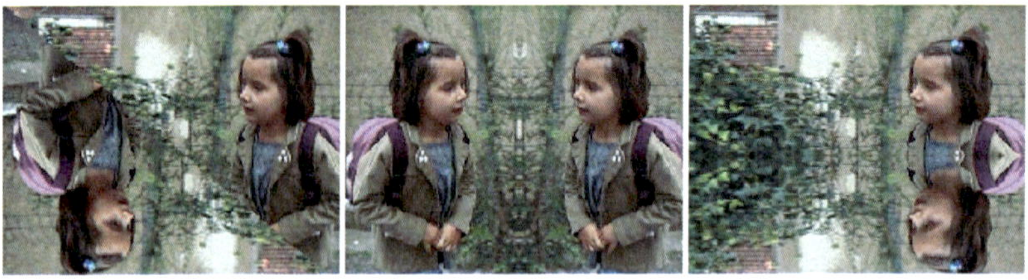

What do you see?

When I look in the mirror, I see a middle-aged guy, with thinning hair (and I'm being generous), with lines and wrinkles and puffy eyes and imperfections everywhere; the products of age and abuse.

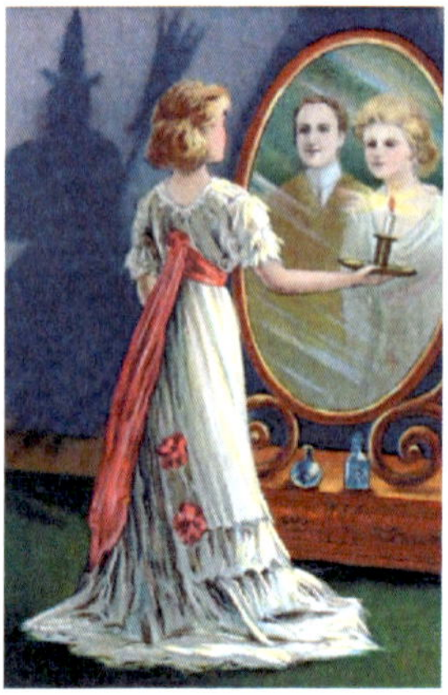

You're perfect! Everything is wonderful!

In other words, I'm looking good! I'm fabulous! I'm megahot! I'm the bomb!

Back to you. Are you not beautiful, elegant; the perfect lady? (For women)

Or handsome, debonair, refined; the perfect gentleman? (For men)

I think you are fabulous because you are reading my book. In fact, I'm sure of it.

So it's agreed then, you're great. And since it's all about you, let's find out why you are so important to the world. On second thought, let's expand our range of your kingdom, to the universe. If there are multiple universes, you're on your own.

There are all sorts of people, but I've never met someone who didn't want to be important. Which does not in any way imply that if we are meek or humble, we cannot be important too. It's just more difficult a state of being to achieve. For instance, in 1997, two examples of important, yet dissimilar, people made the news when they died: Mother Teresa and Princess Diana.

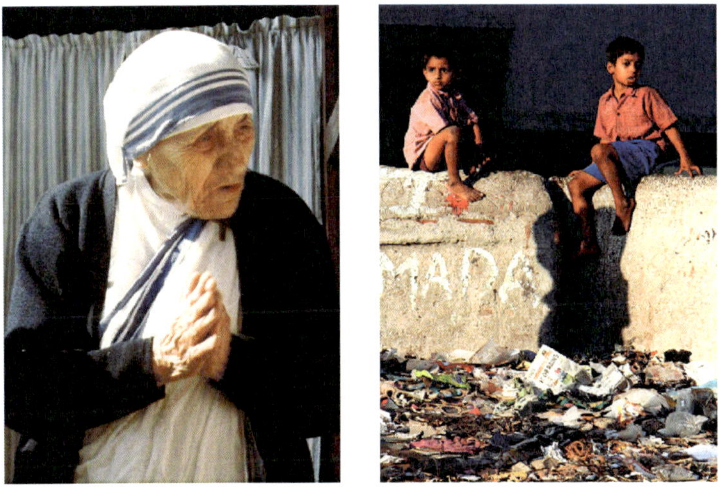

A living Saint and the poor she sacrificed for.

Mother Teresa was a modern Saint. She won the Nobel Peace prize, for a life of extraordinary service to the poorest and most destitute people in the world, the lowest caste members of Indian society, considered by some to be human garbage. The smell of the poor and sick is by itself a difficult thing to endure. Add to that disease, infections, wasting, purulent secretions, and you have a scene out of Dante's Inferno. Now imagine not only taking care of these suffering creatures and not leaving to go home to a comfortable house and well-stocked pantry. Imagine living with them for fifty years, eating what they eat, sleeping on the floor, suffering with the poor in every imaginable way.

For the love of Jesus she did these things. For in her way of living, she was trying to come closer to God. Closer to Him, meant closer to spiritual perfection, which was her way of expressing His love for the world.

Two things she said have never left me: "Do small things with great love" and "We are not here to be successful, we are here to be faithful."

Even this wonderful woman was impatient and rigid at times. These venial sins not withstanding, what she achieved, in this horrible world, ever tested by the demons of doubt, was the one thing that consumed her: Being God's loyal servant.

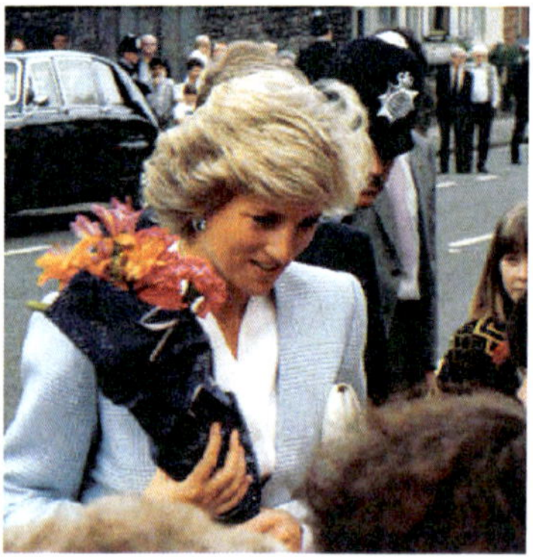

Princess Diana engaging in one of many charitable works.

Now to another important person, Princess Diana. One might consider her an icon for secular humanism. She was a beautiful Princess with an ability to communicate on a spiritual level with millions of people, who were touched by her persona. She led an effort to clean up mine fields so kids wouldn't be blown up, or crippled, and led many other humanitarian efforts to make the world a better place. I think there was also something missing in her life that made her beloved by many, a certain insecurity, and vulnerability, which helped people feel closer to her, and appreciate her.

But what about you and me? How can we possibly compete with such eminent figures, to become important like them?

The answer is that we don't have to do anything extraordinary to be important, we just think we do.

All you need to do is your best! If you consider how simple that is, you won't be so concerned about your place in the Universe. For from a distance of a zillion light years, with all of eternity to work on us, to shape and reshape us like a potter, God will probably cut us some slack. For when He created the world and universe, He never said it was super, great, fantastic, or most excellent. The best He could offer as a "grade" was good and very good! Now if the Creator of the Universe can live with very good, why can't we?

From the earliest time, Biblically speaking, it's always been about failure and triumph (the order is intentional). Call it what you want, as soon as man and woman wanted too much, as in Original Sin, as my Christian brethren believe, things have been interesting. As in the clever Chinese curse, "May you have an interesting life." In my way of thinking, God set Adam and Eve up, for the "fall", and theologians should call it "Original Blaming." For, in a free-for-all of He said, he said, she said, everyone (except for the Serpent), passed on the blame. And it was exit stage left, this way to the egress, for Adam and Eve and their Garden party. And things have never been the same.

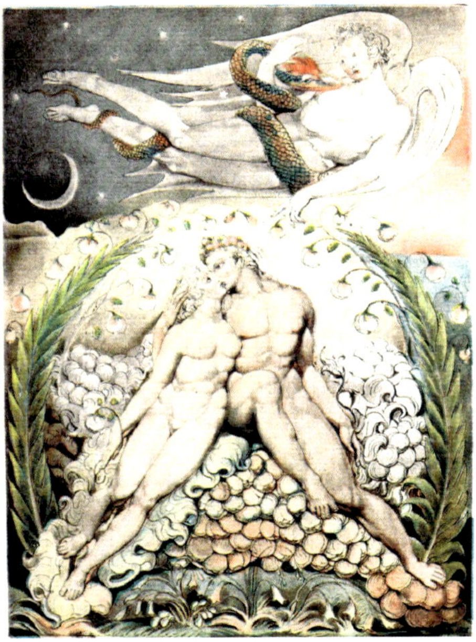

A William Blake image of Satan with Adam and Eve. Wait 'til God finds out!

But in so doing, God added to the complexity of being human, and free will may be one of His greatest gifts. Perhaps the freedom to do our best is the most important element to being important!

So knock yourself out, with acts of kindness, and love, in the smallest of ways, and maybe someday people will be writing about you!

Acknowledgements

I am grateful to many people for various reasons:

My dear mother, Pearl, who taught me to love to read. My late father, Bernie, who demonstrated a certain consistency and work ethic. My brother, Ronald, who is worldly and capable of doing amazing things. My uncle, Mr. Stanley Buchholtz, who is a great role model and inspiration.

My beautiful wife, Victoria, who taught me to say: "I love you." My sons Zachariah and Jacob who have been such a blessing, showing great maturity at times, beyond their years, and a wonderful spirit.

My scientific and medical mentors, all men of great achievement, who taught me so much:

Dr. Alfred Pfister, Dr. Neil Cornell, Dr. Luiz Travassos, Dr. Kenneth Lloyd, Dr. Hiroshi Shiku, Dr. William Voelter, Dr. Ron Christianson, Dr. Wolfgang Dahnert, Dr. Edward Barylak, and Dr. Lloyd Old.

Special thanks to Dr. Ferdy Lejeune, Dr. Yvonne Saenger, Dr. Jedd Wolchok, and Dr. Robert Schreiber, along with their colleagues, for their kind permission to use images from the online journal, Cancer Immunity, which is one of Dr. Old's many innovative creations. I strongly encourage interested readers to visit the Cancer Immunity website www.cancerimmunity.org, which is free to the public and includes a wealth of information on cancer immunology from some of the world's leading scientists and clinicians.

Most of the other images were obtained through the public domain sites of Wikipedia (and its associated search engines, Wikipedia Commons and Mayflower), the National Library of Medicine, and the National Cancer Institute, and we are extremely grateful to all the contributors who have participated in this process. The list of credits, references, and sources is as accurate as possible, but I apologize if anyone was left out, and also apologize, and am responsible for any errors that may have occurred in the preparation of this manuscript.

Nancy Leyrer, Dr. Old's loyal assistant, and Mr. Dan Loos, Esq. both of whom provided encouragement and ideas.

My superb and loyal nurses and staff over many years: Judy Petz, RN, Kate Newbanks, RN, Dianne Haszel, RN, Janet Miller, RN, and Trish Mayhew, RN.

Terri and Todd Engle helped a great deal in the early manuscript preparation; Nance Natelle was instrumental in honing the book to publication quality. Mr. Mark Richter should receive special credit for his tireless efforts in manuscript design and many other areas of artistic input.

The late Mr. Robert Lasdon was a constant source of encouragement throughout a friendship that spanned 35 years.

All the dogs we have loved and have touched our lives, over many years, in the greatest of ways, including Prince, Girlie, Pharoah, Freckles, Hildegarde, Honey, Oprah, Annie, Bianca, and Lima.

My Grandpa, Mr. Charles Buchholtz, who has long passed, but still lives in my heart and mind, and who helped me believe in God.

Above all others, Dr. Barb Natelle, PhD deserves the greatest praise. She is a true friend, whom I love dearly, and I am forever indebted to her.

References

1. Genesis 49:22-24.
2. Beer, et al; Cancer 2007 Oct 25 (Epub).
3. Garland, et al; Am J Public Health 2006 96:252.
4. Abbas, et al; Carcinogenesis 2007 Oct 31 (Epub).
5. Ingraham, et al; Curr Med Res Opin 2007 Nov 21 (Epub).
6. Mohr, et al; J Epidemiol Community Health 2008 62:69.
7. Lindblad-Toh, K., et al; Nature (2005) 438:803.
8. Bergman, PJ, et al; Vaccine (2006) 24:4582.
9. Baxter, et al; Lancet 2005:1054.
10. Levine, et al; Cancer Cell 2005:387.
11. Hohenstein and Fodde; Hum Mol Genet (2003) Epub Aug 5.
12. Hall, et al; Science 1990 250:1684.
13. Putrol, et al; 2006 Drug News Perspect. 19:317.
14. Feng, et al; 2006 Cell 127:621.
15. Cancer Immunity (2004) 5: Suppl 1.
16. Chan, et al; New England Journal of Medicine, Vol 356:2131, 2007.
17. Rous, P.; J Exp Med (1911) 13:397.
18. Moertel, et al; N Eng J Med, (1982) 306:201.
19. Ernst; Brit Med J, (2006) 333:1282.
20. Mengs; Anticancer Res, (2002) 22:1399 Ref. 1)
21. Bowman, et al; J Surg Res 2007 142:275.
22. Shin and Rosen; Arch Pathol Lab Med 2002 126 :697.
23. Stanford Univ Cancer Ctr Website: Breast Cancer (LCIS) info.
24. Aulmann, et al; Breast Cancer Res Treat 2007 Mar 23 (Epub).
25. Shelley Hwang, et al; Cancer 2004 100:2562.
26. Gross, L; Blood (1954) Vol 9 No 6 pgs. 557-573.
27. Arenberger, et al; (2008) J Acad Dermat Venereol 22:56.
28. Ranieri, et al; (2005) Plast Reconstr Surg 115:1058.
29. Visus, et al; Mel Res (2007) 17:83.
30. Denninghoff, et al; Mol Diagn (2004) 8:253 1).
31. Storrs, et al; Science, 183:851, 1974.
32. Luke 7:12-19.

33. New York Times 2/21/06 Nicholas Wade: "Stem Cells May be Key to Cancer".
34. Ramer and Hinz; J Natl Cancer Inst 2007 Dec 25 (Epub).
35. Munson, et al; J Natl Cancer Inst 1975 55:597.
36. Guzman, et al; Br J Cancer 2006 95:197.
37. Preet, et al; Oncogene 2007 Jul 9 (Epub).
38. Hart, et al; Cancer Res 2004 64:1943.

Images, Diagrams, and Photographs

The credits for all images, diagrams, and photographs are to the best of my knowledge correctly attributed, and either within the popular domain or obtained with the authors permission. Any errors are my own, and if any inaccuracies have occurred, we welcome the interested readers' corrections.

Credit numbers for each page are listed starting in the top left-hand corner and read left to right, in the same descending order.

Cover: Courtesy of the National Library of Medicine
(NLM) #A024304
Title: Cancer the Killer
Springfield, ILL Dept of Public Health, [1925]

Page facing Preface: Courtesy NLM #B029693
Title: Famous French Clinician, Professor A. Borrel, MD
Artist: H. Frantz

Essay I

pg. 2	Courtesy: NLM Title: Vaincre le Cancer Author: Bernard Villemot (1911-) Ligue nationale francaise contre le cancer
pg. 2	Courtesy: NLM Title: Le Cancer Peut Etre, Queri s'il est Traite a Son Debut. [1945?] Author: Andre Wilquin (1899-) Ligue Francaise Contre le Cancer
pg. 3	Courtesy: NLM #A028050 Title: Cell Wars; Forces Against Cancer (1970) Author: California Museum of Science and Industry
pg. 4	Courtesy: NLM Title: Depistee a Temps, Toute Tumeur est Guerissable (19--) Author: France Ministere de la sante publique et de la population.

Essay II

pg. 5	Courtesy: Wikipedia Commons (WC) Title: Obverse of United States One Dollar Bill, Series 2003
pg. 6	Courtesy: WC Title: President Lyndon B. Johnson Signing the Medicare Bill with (Former Pres.) Harry Truman, July 30,1965 Author: White House Press Office
pg. 6	Courtesy: (W) Title: Centers for Medicare and Medicaid Services Logo Author: U.S. Government
pg. 7	Courtesy: (W) Title: Saint Basil's Cathedral Author: Mr. David Crawshaw

pg. 7 Courtesy: (W)/Vatican Pontificate
Title: Constantine's Baptism
Author: Fresco Stanze di Constantin Palazzi

Essay III

pg. 8 Courtesy: Dr. Ferdy Lejeune/ Cancer Immunity Journal
Source: Cancer Immunity 6:6 (2006); Fig 9
Author: Dr. Ferdy Lejeune

pg. 9 Courtesy: Dr. Ferdy Lejeune/ Cancer Immunity Journal
Source: Cancer Immnity 6:6 (2006); Fig. 8
Author: Dr. Ferdy Lejeune

pg. 9 Courtesy: (W)
Title: Cartilage Polarised
Author: Emmanuelm (talk)

pg. 10 Courtesy: (WC)
Title: Chondrosarcoma (4)
Author: Unknown

pg. 10 Courtesy: (WC)
Title: Chondrosarcoma (1)
Author: Unknown

pg. 11 Courtesy: (W)
Title: Doxorubicin-3d-Sticks
Author: Sbrools

pg. 11 Courtesy: (W)
Title: Ifosfamide
Author: Dr. Andel Fruh

pg. 11 Courtesy: (W)
Title: GMCSF Crystal Structure
Author: Dr. D.A. Rozwarski et al
Source: Proteins vol. 26 p 304-313 (1996)

pg. 12 Courtesy: (WC)
Title: Macs Killing Cancer Cell
Author: Ms. Susan Arnold
Source: Dr. Rawf Guirguis
Image id 2370, National Cancer Institute

pg. 13 Courtesy: (WC)
Title: Assyrian Horse Archer (8th century BC)
Author: Unknown

pg. 13 Courtesy (W)
Title: Palnetoki
Author: Jenny Nystrom (1854-1946)
Source: Ekermamm A. (1895)
Fran Nordens forntid: Fornnordiska sagor
bearb svenska

Essay IV

pg. 14 Courtesy: (WC)
Title: Squamous Cell Carcinoma
Author: Unlnowm
Source: National Cancer Institute

pg. 14 Courtesy: (WC)
Title: Basaliom3
Author: Mr. Josef Wienand

pg. 15 Courtesy: National Library of Medicine
#A028213
Title: You Can Help Defeat Cancer [1984]
Author: Singapor Ministry of Health, Training
& Health Education Dept.

Essay V

pg. 16 Courtesy: (WC)
Title: Inset Codfish Map
Author: Herman Moll c. 1654

pg. 16 Courtesy: (W)
Title: Codstamp (Newfoundland)
Author: Jcmurphy

pg. 17 Courtesy: (WC)
Title: Cholesterol
Author: NEUROtiker

pg. 17 Courtesy: (WC)
Title: Cholecaliferol 2
Author: NEUROticker

pg. 17 Courtesy: (WC)
Title: Calcitriol 2
Author: NEUROtiker

pg. 18 Courtesy: (WC)
Title: Cold Shower (1898)
Author: Georgios Iakovidis (1853-1932)

Essay VI

pg. 19 Courtesy: (WC)
Title: Troubezkoy Friends (1901)
Author: Paolo Troubezkoy

pg. 19 Courtesy: (WC)
Title: Watchdog of the Treasury, 1800 Seal
Author: U.S. Dept. of the Treasury

pg. 20 Courtesy: (WC)
Title: Balto
Author: Unknown

pg. 20 Courtesy: (WC)
Title: Belka and Strelka Russian Space Dogs

pg. 20 Courtesy: (WC)
Title: POL COA Pobog
Author: S. Voytek based on template by Bastianow which is based on works of Mr. Tadeusz Gajl

pg. 20 Courtesy: (WC)
Title: Blason Ville Adelange (Moselle)
Author: Blazon Project/ ZEFOX

pg. 20 Courtesy: (WC)
Title: Blason Famille La Varenne
Author: Manassas/ Blazon Project

pg. 21 Courtesy: (WC)
Title: Canine Malignant Melanoma
Author: Caroldermoid

pg. 22 Courtesy: (WC)
Title: Boone, Hunter & Dog
Author: David McConeghy

Essay VII

pg. 23 Courtesy: (WC)
Title: 057 Cracow
Author: Rj 979

pg. 23 Courtesy: (WC)
Title: Astronomische Uhr Wells
Author: Aleister Crowley

pg. 23 Courtesy: (WC)
Title: Al- Jazari; A Candle Clock
Author: Farruk ibn Abd al-Latif

pg. 23 Courtesy: (WC)
Title: Al- Jazari Automata; Elephant Clock 1315
Author: Farkh ibn Abd al-Latif

pg. 24 Courtesy: (WC)
Title: Northshield Court 2007-05-27
Author: Jonathunder

pg. 24 Courtesy: (WC)
Title: SCA Combat Example
Author: Unknown

pg. 25 Courtesy: (WC)
Title: Graenfoour
Author: Joan Porunn

pg. 25 Courtesy: (WC)
Title: Four-leaf clover
Author: Phyzome

pg. 25 Courtesy: (WC)
Title: Red Clover (NGM XXXI p516)

pg. 25 Courtesy: (WC)
Title: Warfarin
Author: Calvero

pg. 26 Courtesy: (WC)
Title: RAS Pig01
Author: T Taylor

pg. 26 Courtesy: (WC)
Title: Heparin-3D-structures
Author: Benjah-bmm27

pg. 26 Courtesy: (WC)
Title: Leech–China
Author: Shizhao

pg. 26 Courtesy: (WC)
Title: Hirudin In Complex With Thrombin
Author: Tischler from T.J. Rydel et al Sceience v.249, S277 (1990)

pg. 27 Courtesy: (WC)
Title: Janus Coin
Author: DieBuche

pg. 28 Courtesy: (WC)
Title: Surgical Instruments
Author: John of Arderne from Mirror of Phlebotomy & Practice of Surgery c. 1425-1550

pg. 28 Courtesy: (WC)
Title: Bloodletting 276Px
Author: from S. Noyes/ Hans von Gersdorff: Felduch der Wundarznei 1517

pg. 28 Courtesy: (WC)
Title: Medical Zodiac-Man
Author: John of Arderne from Mirror of Phlebotomy & Practice of Surgery c. 1425-1550

Essay VIII

pg. 29 Courtesy: (WC)
Title: Angel Inurria
Author: Rafael Jimenez

pg. 29 Courtesy: (WC)
Title: BRCA Genes-Location of BRCA1 and BRCA2 On Chromosomes 13 and 17.gif
Author: Kevin Saff

pg. 30 Courtesy: (W)
Title: Breast Cancer
Author: Emmanuelm

pg. 30 Courtesy: (WC)
Title: Cancer
Author: Alessio Govi
Source: Uranographia, Johann Bode

pg. 31 Courtesy: (WC)
Title: Mendel Gregor 1822-1884
Author: Inconnu
Source: The History of Biology de Erik Nordenskiold Ed, Knopf 1928

pg. 31 Courtesy: (WC)
Title: Mendel Seven Characters
Author: Mariana Ruiz Lady of Hats
Source: Molecular Cell Biology: James Darnell

pg. 31 Courtesy: (WC)
Title: Doperwt rijserwt peulen Pisum
Author: Dopert rijserwt peulen

pg. 32 Courtesy: (WC)
Title: Monkey-typing
Author: Brim

pg. 33 Courtesy: (WC)
Title: Oocyte Graulosa Cell
Author: RWJ MS IVF Laboratory/ Ekem

pg. 33 Courtesy: (WC)
Title: Macrophage ARF
Author: Inconspicuo
Source: Inman M. PLOS Biology vol.4/6/2006 e190 Inconspicuous Consumption: Uncovering the Molecular Pathways Behind Phagocytosis

pg. 33 Courtesy: (WC)
Title: Spindle Centriole- Embryonic Brain Mouse-TEM
Authors: Louisa Howard and Miguel Marin-Padilla

pg. 33 Courtesy: (WC)
Title: Leukemia Cells That Contain Epstein Barr Virus Using a FA Staining Technique PHIL 2984 /ores
Author: Dr. Paul M. Feorino/CDC

pg. 33 Courtesy: (WC)
Title: Andromeda Action Core
Author: NASA, ESA & A. Schaller

pg. 33 Courtesy (WC)
Title: Ewing Sarcoma Cells
Author: Lance Liotta Laboratory
Source: PLOS Biology vol 3/8/2005, e276
Cancer Causing Genes Can Convert Even the Most Committed Cells

pg. 33 Courtesy: (WC)
Title: Toxoplasma Gondii
Authors: Ke Hu and John Murray
Source: Hu et al pathogens.plosjoural.org

pg. 33 Courtesy: (WC)
Title: Fluorescent Cells
Author: Unknown
Source: NIH

pg. 33 Courtesy: (WC)
Title: Axopodium Mikrotubuli
Author: Michael Linnenbach

pg. 33 Courtesy: (WC)
Title: Hepatitis A Virus 01
Author: Betty Partin
Source: CDC

pg. 33 Courtesy: (WC)
Title: Galaxy Cluster Roentgen and Gravity Lens
Author: Velko Ruse
Source: NASA

pg. 33 Courtesy: (WC)
Title: Sig06-005
Author: P.N. Appleton
Source: NASA/JPL/SSC/Caltech

pg. 34 Courtesy: (W)
Title: VEGF Receptors
Author: Mikael Haggstrom

pg. 34 Courtesy: NLM
Title: Joshua Lederberg
Source: NIH

pg. 34	Courtesy: (WC) Title: God Dividing Light From Darkness Author: Michelangelo-Sistine Chapel 1509 Source: Web Gallery of Art
pg. 34	Courtesy: (WC) Title: Kirche: Diagram of the Names of God Author: Athanasius Kircher Source: Oedipus Aegyptiacus
pg. 34	Courtesy: (WC) Title: God-Dice Author: John Reid

Essay IX

pg. 35	Courtesy: Elephantiasis Pictures Title: Scrotal Elephantiasis Source: elephantiasis.freeyellow.com/eleph -fiji.gif
pg. 35	Courtesy: (W) Title: Elephantiasis Author: Salvadorjo Source: CDC
pg. 35	Courtesy: Elephantiasis Pictures Title: Ascaris Lumricoides (Roundworms) Source: www.spol.com/micro/worms/ imagepages/image/.htm
pg. 36	Courtesy: (W) Title: Adult Caenorhabditis Elegans Author: Kbradnam
pg. 37	Courtesy: (WC) Title: Alfred Nobel Adjusted Author: Gosta Florman (1831-1900)
pg. 37	Courtesy: (WC) Title: RF 00503 Author: Rfam database Source:www.sanger.ac.uk

pg. 37	Courtesy: (WC) Title RF 00044 Author: Rfam database Source: www.sanger.ac.uk
pg. 37	Courtesy: (WC) Title: RF 00126 Author: Rfam database Source:www.sanger.ac.uk
pg. 38	Courtesy: (WC) Title: RNAi Author: Unknown Source: PLOS Biology.org
pg. 38	Courtesy: (WC) Title: Nobel Prize Medal Author: Gusme
pg. 39	Courtesy: (WC) Title: RNA-code AZ-codons Author: Barbarossa
pg. 39	Courtesy: (WC) Title: Macrobius, Universe With the Earth In the Centre Author: Macrobius Ambrosius Theodosius ca.1150

Essay X

pg. 40	Courtesy (WC) Title: Dr Cluny Macpherson; Egypt 1915 Source: Provincial Archives of Newfoundland and Labrador
pg. 41	Courtesy: (WC) Title: Sphinx MET 11.1 85 Source: Metropolitan Museum of Art
pg. 41	Courtesy: WC Title: Gustave Moreau 005 Author: Gustave Moreau 1864 Source: The Yorck Project

pg. 42 Courtesy: (WC)
Title: Cell Membrane Drawing
Author: Dana Burns
Source: M.S. Bretscher: The molecules of the cell membrane Scientific American 1985 v. 253(4) pg. 86-90

pg. 43 Courtesy: Biomedical Beat Cool Image Gallery
Author: Dr. Kathryn Howell - Univ. of Colorado Health Sciences Center
Source: NIH

pg. 44 Courtesy: (WC)
Title: Sphingolipid en
Author: Lennert B
Source: Benutzer Karl Langner

pg. 44 Courtesy: (WC)
Title: N-Acetylneuraminyl-Galactosyl Ceramide
Author: NEUROtiker

pg. 45 Courtesy: (WC)
Title: ABO Blood Group Diagram
Author: InvictaHOG

Essay XI

pg. 47 Courtesy: (WC)
Title: Old-Woman-Shoe
Author: Nichal p

pg. 47 Courtesy: (WC)
Title: Rosette (Broguing)
Author: Rainer Ersfeld

pg. 48 Courtesy: (WC)
Title: DSCN 1386
Author: Nrbelex

pg. 49 Courtesy: (WC)
Title: Blue Betta Fish Super Delta
Author: Dvortygirl

pg. 49 Courtesy: (WC)
Title: Valle-Inclan
Author: Joseluis bn
Source: Ramon del Valle-Inclan (1866-1936)

pg. 49 Courtesy: (WC)
Title: Pacman Frog
Author: Grosscha

pg. 50 Courtesy: (W)
Title: Monoclonal Ab
Author: Ramujana
Source P. Carter: Improving the efficacy of antibody-based cancer therapies Nat Rev Cancer 2001; 1:118-129

pg. 51 Courtesy: Dr. Robert D. Schreiber
Title: The Three Es of Cancer Immunoediting
Source: Cancer Immunity, Vol. 5 Suppl. 1 (6 April 2005)

pg. 52 Courtesy: (WC)
Title: Manahattan Night March USA
Author: diasUndkompott
Source: Flckr asfilm2-21

pg. 52 Courtesy: (WC)
Title: USS-Akron-Manhattan
Author: Unknown
Source: US Naval historical Center

Essay XII

pg. 53 Courtesy: (WC)
Title: Hippokrates
Author: Polarlys
Source: Baumeister Denkmaler des Klassischen Alterums 1885

pg. 53 Courtesy: (WC)
Title: Hippocratic Oath
Author: Rmrfstar
Source: Ira M. Rutkow, MD; page 27: Surgery: An Illustrated History

pg. 54 Courtesy: (WC)
Title: Salix Alba 013
Author: Willow

pg. 54 Courtesy: (WC)
Title: Yew Bark Taxol PD
Author: Catherine Munro
Source: Mike Trumball/NIH

pg. 54 Courtesy: (WC)
Title: Bayer Heroin 1911
Author: Filnik

pg. 55 Courtesy: (WC)
Title: Cox-2 Inhibited by Aspirin
Author: Dr. Jeff Dahl

pg. 55 Courtesy: (WC)
Title: Aspirin- Structure
Author: Sverdrup

Essay XIII

pg. 56 Courtesy: Bagel Oasis
Title: Poppy Seed Bagel
Author: Unknown

pg. 56 Courtesy: (WC)
Title: Neanderthal 2D
Author: Ivan Lanin

pg. 56 Courtesy: (W)
Title: Our Brun Parcanimal-Ierpyrenees
Jean-noel Lafarque

pg. 57 Courtesy: (WC)
Title: Opium Poppy
Author: Honza XJ

pg. 57 Courtesy: (WC)
Title: Opium Poppy Mohnkapsel
Author: Schlonz?Superfantastic
Source: Flickr

pg. 57 Courtesy: (WC)
Title: Poppy Seeds
Author: Odedr

pg. 58 Courtesy: (WC)
Title: Morphine
Author: Unknown

pg. 58 Courtesy: (WC)
Title: Heroin-Heroine
Author: NEUROtiker

pg. 58 Courtesy: (WC)
Title: Codeine
Author: Unknown

pg. 58 Courtesy: (WC)
Title: Methodon
Author: Unknown

pg. 59 Courtesy: (W)
Title: Morphine Advertisement 1900
Author: Mike C line
Source: Overland Monthly; January 1906

pg. 59 Courtesy: (W)
Title: Bayer Heroin Bottle
Author: Mpv-51

pg. 59 Courtesy: (W)
Title: Opium Eater
Author: Unknown
Source: Penguin Books

pg. 59 Courtesy: Johns Hopkins Medical Archives
Title: Mrs. William Halstead (Caroline Hampton)
Source: Halstead- Photo Gallery

pg. 59 Courtesy: Johns Hopkins Medical Archives
Title: Dr. Halstead in Surgery
Source: Halstead-Photo Gallery

pg. 60 Courtesy: Johns Hopkins Medical Archives
Title: Dr. William Halstead
Source: Halstead-Photo Gallery

Essay XIV

pg. 61 Courtesy: NIH
Title: Sanguine
Source: NLM

pg. 61 Courtesy: NIH
Title: Melancholy
Source: NLM

pg. 61 Courtesy: NIH
Title: Phlegmatic
Source: NLM

pg. 61 Courtesy: NIH
Title: Choleric
Source: NLM

pg. 62 Courtesy: (WC)
Title: Recurrent Breast Cancer
Author: Kauczuk

pg. 63 Courtesy: (WC)
Title: Religious Syms
Author: Rursus
Source: Stalik/ Manup

pg. 63 Courtesy: (WC)
Title: Major World Religious Pictures
Author: Nyo

pg. 63 Courtesy: NIH
Title: William Osler, MD
Source: NLM

pg. 63 Courtesy: NIH
Title: William Osler, MD
Source: NLM

pg. 65 Courtesy: NIH
Title: The Workes of That Famous Chirugion Ambrose Parey
Author: Tho. Johnson
Source: NLM

pg. 65 Courtesy: (W)
Title: Ambroise Pare
Author: William Holl (1807-1871)

Essay XV

pg. 67 Courtesy: (WC)
Title: Flight of Lot
Author: Gustave Dore

pg. 70 Courtesy (WC)
Title: Australian Infantry Small Box Respirators
Author: Capatain Frank Hurley
Source: Australian War Memorial

pg. 70 Courtesy: (W)
Title: Mustard Gas Burns
Author: Unknown
Source: Library & Archives Canada

pg. 70 Courtesy: (WC)
Title: Doktorschnabel 430px
Author: Paul Furst
Source: NLM

pg. 70 Courtesy: (WC)
Title: Dog With Mask WWI
Author: Frank Whiting Halsey
Source: The Literary Digest; History of the World War, volume V p. 333 (1920)

pg. 70 Courtesy: (WC)
Title: Small Box Respirator
Author: Simon Jones, World War I Gas Warfare Tactics and Equipment, Osprey Publishing 2007
Source: Imperial War Museum

pg. 71 Courtesy: (W)
Title: Estramustine
Author: Unknown

pg. 71 Courtesy: (W)
Title: Melphalan
Author: Unknown

pg. 71 Courtesy: (W)
Title: Mechlorethamine
Author: Unknown

pg. 72 Courtesy: (W)
Title: Herceptin Fab
Author: Py Mol

pg. 73 Courtesy: (WC)
Title: Apocalypse Vasnetsov
Author: Victor Vasenetov 1887
Source: http//ljrosia.org/users/johnpetrov/
166993html

Essay XVI

pg. 74 Courtesy: (W)
Title: Payton Manning
Author: Cpl. Michelle M. Dickson, USMC

pg. 74 Courtesy: (W)
Title: Ted Geisel NYWTS
Author: Al Ravenna, World Telegram staff photographer
Source: U.S. Library of Congress

pg. 75 Courtesy: Nobelprize.org
Title: Payton Rous
Author: Nobel Foundation

pg. 75 Courtesy: (WC)
Title: Cowboy
Author: J.C.H. Grabill; Sturgis, Dakota Terr. c.1888
Source: U.S. Library of Congress

pg. 75 Courtesy: (WC)
Title: Buffalo Bill Wild West Show c 1899
Author: Unknown
Source: U.S. Library of Congress

pg. 76 Courtesy: (WC)
Title: Cock El Bolson
Author: Fabien Khan

pg. 76 Courtesy: (WC)
Title: Rabbit Shopes Papilloma Virus 3
Author: WD 45
Source: http//flickr.com/photos/wd45/

pg. 77 Courtesy: (WC)
Title: Smallpox Virus
Authors: Fred Murphy & Sylvia Whitfield
Source: CDC

pg. 77 Courtesy: (WC)
Title: Smallpox Vaccine
Author: Unknown
Source: CDC

pg. 77 Courtesy: (WC)
Title: Poster For Vaccination Against Small Pox
Author: Unknown
Source: CDC

pg. 77 Courtesy: (WC)
Title: A Nurse Holding a Young Child
Author: Vila, artist 1917
Source: U.S. Library of Congress

Essay XVII

pg. 78 Courtesy: (W)
Title: Amygdalin
Author: Unknown

pg. 79 Courtesy: (WC)
Title: Apricot Tree
Author: Fir 0002

pg. 79 Courtesy: (WC)
Title: Jaws Great White Shark South Australia
Author: Niranjan
Source: http//www.flickr.com/people/9075901@NO2

pg. 79 Courtesy: (WC)
Title: Mistletoe P1210829
Author: David Monniaux

pg. 81 Courtesy: (WC)
Title: Alternative Juice
Author: Unknown

pg. 81 Courtesy: (WC)
Title: Kickapoo Sagwa
Author: Unknown

pg. 81 Courtesy: (WC)
Title: Ayers Cathartic Pills
Author: Unknown
Source: S merdis of Tlon

pg. 81 Courtesy: (WC)
Title: Pink Pills for Pale People
Author: Unknown
Source: Smerdis of Tlon

pg. 81 Courtesy: (WC)
Title: Peruvian Wine of Coca
Author: Unknown

pg. 81 Courtesy: (WC)
Title: Radam's Microbe Killer
Author: Unknown

pg. 83 Courtesy: (WC)
Title: Cebocap
Authors: Elaine and Arthur Shapiro
Source: NIH

pg. 83 Courtesy: (WC)
Title: AntiLirium Placebo
Authors: Elaine and Arthur Shapiro
Source: NIH

pg. 83 Courtesy: (WC)
Title: Four Placebs
Authors: Elaine and Arthur Shapiro
Source: NIH

Essay XVIII

pg. 84 Courtesy: (WC)
Title: Mammo Breast Cancer
Author: Unknown
Source: NCI

pg. 85 Courtesy: NLB
Title: A Medical Consultation
Author: Unknown
Source: order# A022030

pg. 85 Courtesy: (WC)
Title: Normal
Author: Itayba

pg. 85 Courtesy: (WC)
Title: Breast DCIS Histopathology (1)
Author: Unknown

pg. 85 Courtesy: (WC)
Title: Breast Invasive Lobular Carcinoma (1)
Author: KGH

pg. 85 Courtesy: (WC)
Title: Intraductal Papilloma Histopathology (2)
Smooth Muscle Actin
Author: KGH

pg. 85 Courtesy: NLM
Title: Finding a Breast Cancer Tumor Can be Like Finding a Needle In a Haystack
Author: Bethesda, MD Medical Arts and Photography Branch, 199-?
Source: Order# C00243

Essay XIX

pg. 86 Courtesy: (WC)
Title: Light Switch Inside Explained
Author: Scott Ehardt

pg. 86 Courtesy: (WC)
Title: Bombeta de Llum
Author: Unknown

pg. 86 Courtesy: (WC)
Title: Schuss Gluebirne
Authors: Markus Kempf & Frank Bastian, 1991

pg. 87 Courtesy: (WC)
Title: Sequent Calculus for Classical Libnear Logic
Author: Kaustuv Chaudhuri, 2004

pg. 87 Courtesy: (WC)
Title: Vector Field
Author: Fibonacci, 2007

pg. 89 Courtesy: (WC)
Title: Thorax CT Peripheres Bronchial-Carcinoma li OF
Author: Lange 123, 2004

pg. 89 Courtesy: (WC)
Title: Mammogram Showing Breast Cancer
Author: Unknown
Source: NIH

pg. 89 Courtesy: (WC)
Title: Anaplastic Astrocytoma
Author: T. Fujmaki et al
Source: Biomed Central License

pg. 90 Courtesy: (WC)
Title: Taenidiael
Author: Dietma Riedel

pg. 90 Courtesy: (WC)
Title: Lung Epithelium 80294-2.6
Authors: Louisa Howard & Michael Binder
Source: Dartmouth College

pg. 90 Courtesy: (WC)
Title: Fortuna or Fortune
Author: (Hans) Sebald Benham (1500-1550)
Source: scan by Yellow Lion 2006

Essay XX

pg. 91 Courtesy: (WC)
Title: Nur 04507
Author: Unknown
Source: National Undersea Research Program

pg. 92 Courtesy: (W)
Title: Ludwik Gross
Author: Unknown (uploaded by user Furfur)
Source: NLM

pg. 92 Courtesy: (WC)
Title: Colourful Thermophilic Archaebacteria Stain In Midway Geyser Basin
Author: Wing- ChiPoon, 2004

pg. 92 Courtesy: (WC)
Title: RT8-4
Author: Xiangyux (Xiaoyu Xiang)

pg. 93	Courtesy: nobelprize.org Title: Kary B. Mullis Source: Nobel Foundation
pg. 93	Courtesy: (WC) Title: PCR Author: Madprime 2007
pg. 93	Courtesy: (WC) Title: PCR Machine2 Author: Magnus Manske
pg. 93	Courtesy: (WC) Title: PCR Tubes Author: Madprime, 2007
pg. 94	Courtesy: (WC) Title: Feline Leukemia Virus Author: Unknown Source: CDC
pg. 96	Courtesy: (WC) Title: Blake: Jacobs Ladder Author: Wiliam Blake (1757-1827)
pg. 96	Courtesy: (WC) Title: Double Helix Nebula-nr6903a Author: Unknown Source: from Audriusa: http//www.spitzer.caltech.edu
pg. 96	Courtesy: (WC) Title: DNA Double Helix 45 Author: Dennis Myts

Essay XXI

pg. 97	Courtesy: Wikipedia Title: Leprosy Author: Arents/Pismire Source: Leloir's atlas on leprosy (1886)
pg. 98	Courtesy: (W) Title: Gerhard Hansen Author: RSabbatini

pg. 98 Courtesy: (W)
Title: M Leprae Ziehl Nielsen 2
Author: Unknown
Source: U.S. Dept of Health and Human Services

pg. 99 Courtesy (WC)
Title: Thalidomide-2D-skeletal
Author: Benjah-bmm 27

pg. 99 Courtesy: (WC)
Title: Thalidomide Baby
Author: Unknown
Source: NCI

pg. 99 Courtesy: (W)
Title: Armadillo
Authors: John and Karen Hollingworth
Source: U.S. Fish and Wildlife Service

pg. 100 Courtesy: (WC)
Title: Multiple Myeloma (1) MG stain
Author: KGH

pg. 100 Courtesy: (W)
Title: Plasmacell
Author: Unknown

Essay XXII

pg. 101 Courtesy: (WC)
Title: Drini-Nonuniform Convergence
Author: Drini

pg. 103 Courtesy: Dr. Yvonne Saenger and Dr. Jedd Wolchok
Title: Response to Ipilmumab Therapy of Patient Case 2
Author: Wolchok et al
Source: Cancer Immunity Journal vol.8:1 (2008); Figure 4

pg. 103 Courtesy: Dr. Yvonne Saenger and Dr. Jedd Wolchok
Title: Response to Ipilmumab Therapy of Patient Case 1
Author: Wolchok et al
Source: Cancer Immunity Journal vol. 8 :1 (2008); Figure 2s

pg. 103 Courtesy: Dr. Yvonne Saenger and Dr. Jedd Wolchok
Title: Response to Ipilmumab Therapy of Patient Case 1
Author: Wolchok et al
Source: Cancer Immunity Journal vol.8 : 1 (2008); Figure 3

pg. 104 Courtesy: Dr. Armin Bender and colleagues
Title: CT Scan of Patient 15
Author: A. Bender et al
Source: Cancer Immunity Journal vol: 7 : 16 (2007) Figure 3

Essay XXIII

pg. 107 Courtesy: (WC)
Title: PET Scan Image
Author: Raziel

Essay XXIV

pg. 108 Courtesy: (WC)
Title: Illustration Cannabis Sativa O
Author: Kurt Stueber
Source: Dr. Otto Wilhelm Thome

pg. 108 Courtesy: (WC)
Title: 11-OH-THC
Author: Isilanes, 2007

pg. 109 Courtesy: NLM
Title: Tissue Culture Research-NCI
Author: Roy Perry
Source: NIH #A024021

pg. 109 Courtesy: NLM
Title: Large Scale Tissue Culture Growth
Author: V. Taylor
Source: NIH #A023996

pg. 110 Courtesy: NLM
Title: Dedication Ceremonies for Buildings 36 and 37
Author: Unknown
Source: NIH #A014716

pg. 110 Courtesy: NLM
Title: NIH-NCI Research Album 4
Author: Unknown
Source: NIH #A020042

pg. 110 Courtesy: NLM
Title: NLM
Author: Unknown
Source: NIH #A020041

pg. 110 Courtesy: (WC)
Title: Reefer Madness 05
Author: Ibaranoff24

pg. 110 Courtesy: (WC)
Title: Reefer Madness 04
Author: Ibaranoff24

pg. 111 Courtesy: (WC)
Title: A Midnight Modern Conversation
Author: Nick Michael, 2006
Source: William Hogarth (1697-1764)

pg. 111 Courtesy: (WC)
Title: Lilly 96B
Author: Unknown
Source: www.AntiqueCannabisBook.com

pg. 111 Courtesy: (WC)
Title: Cannabis Americana; JL Hopkins B
Author: Arnaudh

Essay XXV

pg. 112 Courtesy: (WC)
Title: Gandhi at the Telephone
Author: Yann
Source: www.mkgandhi.org

pg. 112 Courtesy: (WC)
Title: Communications Men
Author: W. Wolny
Source: National Park Service

pg. 112 Courtesy: (WC)
Title: A Telephone Operator
Author: Bubamara
Source: Library of Congress

pg. 112 Courtesy: (WC)
Title: Alexander Graham Telephone In New York
Author: Gilbert H. Grosnevor Collection
Source: Library of Congress

pg. 115 Courtesy: (WC)
Title: Call Waiting
Author: Storker
Source: Flickr

pg. 115 Courtesy: (WC)
Title: Peter Treveris- Engraving of Trepanantion for Handyworke of Surgeri, 1525
Author: Peter Treveris
Source: English Woodcuts 1480-1535; by Edward Hodnett, Oxford University Press, 1973

Essay XXVI

pg. 116 Courtesy: (WC)
Title: Holbein-Death
Author: Michael Wolgemut, 1493

pg. 116 Courtesy: (WC)
Title: Nuremberg Chronicles fllrl
Author: Hartmann Schedel, 1493

pg. 116 Courtesy: (WC)
Title: Michaelangelo Mose 2007
Author: Ulrich Mayring
Source: Michaelangelo

pg. 116 Courtesy: (WC)
Title: Dore Bible; Joseph Makes Himself Known to His Brethren
Author: Rageoss
Source: Gustave Dore

pg. 117 Courtesy: (WC)
Title: Grandma Moses NYWTS
Author: Roger Higgins; NY Word-Telegram and the Sun; Staff Photographer
Source: Library of Congress

pg. 118 Courtesy: NLM
Title: Only X-ray-Rradium-Surgery-Ever Cured Cancer
Author: Fellnagel
Source: U.S. Public Health Service [19--], #A031109

pg. 119 Courtesy: (WC)
Title: Earth Mars Comparison
Author: Unknown
Source: Jet Propulsion Lab/ NASA

pg. 119 Courtesy: (WC)
Title: Gnome Globe Current Event
Author: David Vignoni, Anomie 2007

pg. 119 Courtesy: (WC)
Title: Benzo-a-pyrene Chemical Structure
Author: en:user:cacycle

pg. 119 Courtesy: (WC)
Title: Papilloma Virus (HPV)
Author: Unknown
Source: NCI- Laboratory of Tumor Virus Biology

pg. 119 Courtesy: (WC)
Title: Human Chromosomes Chromomycin A3
Author: Steffen Dietzel, 2006

pg. 119 Courtesy: (WC)
Title: Choroidplexuscarcinoma
Author: Martin Haselblatt, MD, 2006

pg. 120 Courtesy: (WC)
Title: Diptheria Vaccination Poster
Author: Lipothymia
Source: http://www.nationalarchives.gov.uk

pg. 120 Courtesy: (WC)
Title: Black Death
Author: Unknown

pg. 120 Courtesy: (WC)
Title: Penicillin PS Aedit
Author: Unknown
Source: NIH

pg. 121 Courtesy: (WC)
Title: SEM Lymphocyte DO11.10
Source: Dr. Triche- NCI, 1976

pg. 121 Courtesy: L.J. Old, MD
Source: Cancer Research Institute

Essay XXVII

pg. 122 Courtesy: (WC)
Title: Diagonal Mirror
Author: Zecas

pg. 122 Courtesy: (WC)
Title: Diagonal Mirror
Author: Zecas

pg. 122 Courtesy: (WC)
Title: Diagonal Mirror
Author: Zecas

pg. 122 Courtesy: (WC)
Title: Halloween-card-mirror-2
Author: Bill Ellis
Source: Lucifer Ascending: The Occult in Folklore and Popular Culture; Univ of Kentucky, 2004; ISBN 0-8131-2289-9

pg. 123 Courtesy: (WC)
Title: Mother Teresa
Author: Evert Odekerken, 1988

pg. 123 Courtesy: (WC)
Title: Two boys in Dharavi
Author: Wen-Yan King
Source: Flickr/NGOmedapt

pg. 124 Courtesy: (WC)
Title: Princess Diana Bristol, 1987
Author: Rick
Source: Flickr

pg. 125 Courtesy: (WC)
Title: Blake, William (English, 1757-1827), 'Satan Watching the Caresses of Adam and Eve.'
Source: Paradise Lost, 1808; Museum of Fine Arts, Boston, U.S.

Credits for the back book cover images:

Courtesy: NLM
Title: The Sad Story of My Fathers Great Suffering From CANCER
Source: NLM #A012358

Courtesy: NLM
Title: Yoghurt Health News: Cancer Treatment Now Ready
Source: NLM #A012339

Biography

Clifford S. Pukel, MD is a physician who specializes in hematology and oncology. He is a graduate of the University of Miami School of Medicine, completed his internal medicine residency at the University of West Virginia/Charleston Area Medical Center, and subspecialty fellowship at Dartmouth Hitchcock Medical Center.

Prior to his career as a clinician, he was a scientist at Memorial Sloan Kettering Cancer Center working in various areas of research studying cancer cells and the immune response to this disease. His achievements have been recognized, and he has been elected to: Who's Who in the World, America, Science and Engineering, and Medicine and Health Care. He is presently an Assistant Professor of Clinical Medicine at the University of Wisconsin School of Medicine.

After 35 years of both basic research and clinical medicine, this represents his first book. Hopefully his wealth of experience and unique perspective towards the problem of cancer, will lead to other books. He has also created a corporation, the Cancer Immunotherapy Institute, LLC (cancerimmunionst@aol.com) designed to disseminate his ideas and provide funds for the development of new and innovative ways to safely and effectively treat people with cancer.